SLIMMER YOUNGER STRONGER

Lose weight and feel fantastic with tips from the U.S. Olympic team's former trainer!

Imagine how great it would be to wake up every morning full of life and vitality; to bounce out of bed with eagerness and excitement, feeling like a million bucks. *Slimmer, Younger, Stronger* is the key to achieving this goal!

This motivational and practical book provides an easy program that shows you how to incorporate proven health habits into your breathing, eating, sleeping, exercise and thought. Varner presents twelve easy secrets that will help you drop pounds effortlessly, fight aging and disease, increase your energy and concentration and improve your sleep.

Based on sound research, 25 years of proven results and a solid belief in the power of the mind, this program has worked for Olympic gold medalists and non-athletes alike. Its power lies in its simplicity: anyone can improve their health, lose weight and feel more in control with this easy program.

"Incredible! After following the principles in this book,
I lost over 25 pounds and I haven't gained it back. I'm a believer."
_ Ed Crankshaw, *writer, Seaside, CA*

"The 12 principles in this book literally saved my life. I was 86 years old
and needed a walker to get around. Now I'm 96 and lift weights, jog and
do some boxing drills. I feel like I'm a kid again."
_ Mitsuko (Grandma) Bannai,
96-year-old Grandmother, Salt Lake City, UT

"What a fantastic book. The most important aspect is the fact
I am learning how to harness the immense power of my subconscious mind.
Not only am I becoming leaner and healthier,
but I'm improving in other aspects of my life."
_ Ben Leach, *engineer and business consultant, Virginia Beach, VA*

"The most amazing yet the simplest program I've ever done.
I lowered my blood pressure and the breathing program eliminated
my snoring. Excellent book! I wholeheartedly recommend it."
_ Dan Coker, *minister, Glendale, AZ*

"Sam Varner's writing is very easy to understand and very inspiring.
Also, the program really works...thanks, Sam."
_ John Sauer, *strength and conditioning coach,*
College of William and Mary, Williamsburg, VA

"I loved this book. So simple and easy to understand. And it makes sense."
_ Lisa Ragsdale, *administrative assistant, Savannah, GA*

"Sam's approach makes learning about health fun and easy.
The power of prayer and thought make this book complete."
_ Dwight Daub, *CSCS, MS,*
strength and conditioning coach, Seattle Supersonics (NBA)

"This book is a must for anyone who cares about total health and wants to
understand the mind/body connection. I will be using these simple,
make-sense principles and will recommend that others do the same."
_ Jerry Simmons, *head strength and conditioning coach,*
Carolina Panthers (NFL)

"I've known Sam for many years and believe in his health philosophy
and training programs. His research and commitment are evident
in his successes."
_ Scott Mitchell, *former NFL quarterback*

SLIMMER, YOUNGER, STRONGER:

12 Simple Things
You Can Do To Achieve
Optimum Health

SAM VARNER, CSCS

First edition published in hardback in the USA in 2000 by
Element Books, Inc.
160 North Washington Street
Boston, Massachusetts 02114

Published in Great Britain in 2000 by
Element Books Limited
Shaftesbury, Dorset SP7 8BP

Published in Australia in 2000 by
Element Books Limited for
Penguin Books Australia Limited
487 Maroondah Highway, Ringwood, Victoria 3134

Third edition published in softback in the USA in 2005 by
Faith Printing Company
4210 Locust Hill Road
Taylors, South Carolina, 29687

Library of Congress Cataloging-in-Publication data available
British Library Cataloguing in Publication data available

ISBN 0-939241-71-4

Third Edition
10 9 8 7 6 5 4 3

Printed in the United States of America by Faith Printing Co.

Book design by Jill A. Winitzer

Hardback edition - ISBN 1-86204-771-5

I dedicate this book to my beloved father,
Andy C. Varner.
I love you, Pops.

In loving memory of my mother,
the late Hazel P. Varner.
Your love and presence are still felt.

Foreword

Sam Varner is nationally known in the fields of nutrition, health and fitness and currently serves as Director of Living Wellness for The Cliffs Communities. In the following pages, Sam shares a lifetime of knowledge and proven fundamentals for maximizing health and fitness at every level of performance, from amateur to professional. A former trainer of the U.S. Olympic Team and Strength Coach for the 1981-1982 national champion Clemson University football team, Sam has 25 years of experience in providing positive health results for collegiate and professional athletes and for anyone who has shown an interest in self-improvement. Sam has devoted his professional career to helping thousands of people achieve optimal levels of fitness, regardless of age.

Sam's wealth of knowledge stems from his relentless pursuit of research in every aspect of the workings of the human body. From this, he has developed practical approaches to motivate individuals to reach their full potential. He takes this breadth of knowledge and translates his findings in a manner that is easy for readers to understand and implement on a daily basis.

Knowing Sam has had a powerful impact on my life, both personally and in terms of wellness. Not only does Sam coach others in his fundamental health principles, but he lives them as well. Spending time with Sam, I've learned to appreciate his devotion to good health and also his zest for daily life. His spirituality is clearly evident as a part of his overall philosophy.

Sam's book comes at an ideal time. Studies indicate that one of the most significant trends, especially with the baby boomer generation, is to take an active role in preventive health issues while striving to live healthy and long lives. Wellness is important to me on a number of levels. Wellness may be as simple as a sunset hike with neighborhood friends, families sharing a meal, pausing for a quiet moment in nature, or simply a good night's sleep. Wellness is also a part of my core philosophy as a developer.

Sam's expertise has been so inspirational that we've decided to incorporate it as a means of taking wellness a step further for our Cliffs family. We are blessed with the opportunity to expand our premise through a partnership with Sam Varner and his wellness team. It is for many reasons that Sam and his team are the premiere choice for wellness expertise. His comprehensive approach to wellness addresses all aspects of healthy living on physical, mental, emotional and spiritual levels. By combining these approaches, they have brought value to the lives of everyone they touch—individuals from all walks of life

It is my hope that, as you read this book, you too will be inspired by Sam's values to achieve your optimal level of health.

Jim Anthony
The Cliffs Communities

Contents

Acknowledgments

First and foremost, I thank God for the opportunity of sharing my message of health to each and everyone of you. His love and blessings know no bounds.

I give much credit to all the athletes, coaches, trainers and clients whom I have been associated with throughout the years. It is you that have helped shape the scope of this book.

A big thanks to my agent, Nancy Yost, who patiently and successfully coached me through unfamiliar literary waters. More importantly, I sincerely appreciate her faith and belief in me as a writer.

A special thanks to Holly Schmidt, my editor, for her direction, suggestions, insight, and support. Holly's the best.

Thanks to everyone at Element Books for their input, support and all their diligent work in helping me complete this book.

Also, Tony Robbins deserves much gratitude for showing me how to tap my personal power. Tony is a terrific motivator and inspirational role model. Thanks Tony.

I would like to sincerely thank Ed Crankshaw, who initially inspired me to write this book. His ideas and insights about writing made a tremendous difference. Thanks, Ed.

I also appreciate the efforts of Thomas Duckett, Susan Jones, Ken King and Ben Leach for their critique reading and constructive comments.

Much gratitude is owed to Dan Coker and Calvin Turpin for their prayers and spiritual guidance.

Also, thanks to Tom Olivola and David Anderson for the invaluable literary connection.

I commend the Carmel Rotary Club for allowing me to present my material and practice my professional speaking. Thanks also for not falling asleep or throwing anything during my club presentations.

I am also grateful to Lighthouse Baptist Church of Seaside, California, and its Youth Group for their never ending prayers and undying support.

Thanks to Jim Anthony for believing in me and allowing me to be a part of The Cliffs Experience.

Thanks, also, to Topper Hagerman for being the best business partner and friend I could ask for.

Thanks to Kathy Sheppard for her valuable support and endless encouragement.

And lastly, I would like to give a very special thanks to my Dad and Frances and the most adorable Golden Retriever, Raleigh.

Introduction

Imagine how great it would be to wake up every morning full of life and vitality. To bounce out of bed with eagerness and excitement, feeling like a million bucks. How would you like to add years to your life and at the same time enhance the quality of your health? Would you like to reach your ideal body weight and stay there—without dieting? Can you imagine being in the best shape of your life no matter how old you are? What if you could drastically reduce or even eliminate your risks of getting cancer or heart disease merely by implementing a few simple daily habits. In fact, catching a cold or coming down with the flu could be easily minimized or avoided altogether. What would you think if I told you that achieving a leaner, healthier body is as simple as altering your thought process? Well the purpose of this book is quite simply to address these very issues—issues that concern not only your health and well-being but the potentiality of your life.

For the last 25 years I've been on a fervent quest to study and understand the magnificent workings of the human body. During that time I have focused constantly on discovering what makes the human organism tick and how its performance can be maximized. My thirst to learn about optimum health and physical fitness has become unquenchable. The paradigm-shifting information I have discovered throughout my passionate journey can no longer be kept to myself and must be shared with others. It needs to be told because of the amazing impact it could have on many people's lives, including yours. Quite honestly, the material compiled from my experiences and studies may very well save your life or at least positively transform it. To better understand the amazing story, let me first tell you how I started down this very interesting path of discovery.

The year was 1973, and I was just entering my first year of college at North Carolina State University (Go Wolfpack). One of the freshman requirements was to complete a basic physical education class called PE 100. For many of the incoming freshman, this introductory course was merely a class to exercise while receiving college credits. But being one who was never into fitness and never really liked to exercise, I was definitely dreading this mandatory PE course. You see, in high school I didn't have to participate in physical education because I was always involved in the right kind of extracurricular activities that excused me. Well, this was not high school, and I wasn't going to wrangle my way out of this class, which involved weight lifting and jogging. In fact, to pass the course I had to lift a certain amount of weight in a specific lifting exercise and run a mile and a half in a required time.

Early in the course, I grudgingly participated in the required weekly running and weight lifting. At first, I really hated it. But as the semester went by, I surprisingly started to get into the exercise habit. I noticed myself getting stronger, and my slow-paced jogging began to get easier. By the end of the semester when the day came for the timed run and lifting tests, I was ready. The physical tests were tough and challenging but not nearly as difficult as I had originally imagined. What I had dreaded at the start of the semester on that hot August day turned out to be not that difficult after all. As a matter of fact, the class made me feel physically and mentally alive.

From then on, I was hooked! Hooked on exercise. Not only did I engulf myself in a regimented physical fitness program after PE 100, but I began to look more closely at health and the human body. The positive effects of consistent exercise and healthier eating habits on our bodies really fascinated me. In fact, I developed such a passion to learn more about this subject that I even changed my college major from political science to biology. You might say that seemingly simple, insignificant freshman requirement altered the rest of my life. In fact, I went on to receive a degree in biology and also a second BS degree in food science-nutrition. The book you are about to read had its birth from those events in the early 1970s.

My burning thirst to understand more about how to achieve optimum human health continued as I became an aspiring college strength and conditioning coach. Not only did my career involve my life's passion, but in the process I got to work with some of the most elite athletes in the world. All during my 25-year coaching and fitness career I tried to learn as much as I could about human health, while at the same time sharing it with the collegiate and Olympic athletes I was training. However, they had much more than health on their minds; they were focused on achieving maximum performance through whatever means possible. But to me it was all the same. Optimize health and you optimize human performance. The athletes that grasped this concept of optimizing performance through sound, basic health principles were better able to sustain a more successful athletic career.

After I retired from the strength-coaching field, I was asked to assist a few friends who wanted to get into better shape. Little did I know that their ambitions would lead me to a sideline hobby of personal fitness training and then to another career involving my life's passion. The people I was now helping weren't competing for any gold medals, nor were they participating in any NCAA championships or conference crowns. No, the clients I was now involved with just wanted to improve their health, lose a little weight, and generally get more out of the most important game—life. No matter how many different clients I was helping, their fitness goals were universal: to lose body fat and look and feel better.

While successfully working with top-notch athletes and general population clients, I was constantly staying on top of the latest research in the health field, especially nutrition and exercise. It wasn't until recently that I decided to put all my notes, experiences, successes and failures together to create a complete and functional health program. This program entails not only nutrition and exercise, but it incorporates even the more basic elements of health such as sleeping, breathing, an—yes—even the human mind. In fact, the true success of this plan comes from learning how to program your subconscious mind to effectively establish healthy habits and end unwanted ones. This is just one of the many aspects of this book that set it apart from all the other health, fitness and nutritional publications.

In my quest to learn as much about successful human health as I could, I literally read over 500 books, attended countless seminars, and studied hundreds of healthy and successful lifestyles, including the world-class and professional athletes I coached. Throughout all my studies, investigations and experiences, I began to observe the same healthy habits recurring time and again. By identifying these basic tendencies common throughout all my research and experience with top-notch athletes and "regular people"(like you and me), I was able to put together a simple but workable plan. My plan comprises fundamental daily habits and, at the same time, truly addresses the keys to successful living.

People want to know how to lose weight permanently, how to get in shape, how to reduce chances of disease, and how to create the optimum healthy lifestyle. The principles you are about to read will address these questions and much more. And these health principles are as viable for the young, stressed-out career person as they are for the overweight grandmother. This is not a complicated or difficult plan—in fact, many of you are much closer to a fit and healthy body than you might think.

My goal is to help you better understand and hopefully utilize these very valuable principles for a better, longer, more fruitful life.

That's what this book is all about. I have spent years researching practical and scientific material from medical studies to sports medicine, from psychology to anthropology, from nutrition to biochemistry. These pages contain not only solid research but also my experience with some of the nation's top athletes. All the athletes and personal training clients whom I have been involved with for the last 25 years have helped shape the scope of this book. But this is more than a "how to" fitness book. It is a guide to help you reach and maintain the highest pinnacle of physical health and emotional well-being. God intended for everyone to live life to the fullest, and the principles in this book will definitely point you in that direction.

Each chapter of this book details the importance and implementation of five vital health components: breathing, eating, sleeping, exercising and thinking. All of these fundamental principles are presented with extensive research, sound scientific material and basic logic. The end product is a simple, easy to follow, workable plan that includes 12 daily health habits. And since each health principle builds upon the previous one, the 12 habits are listed in descending order, culminating with the anchoring habit in Chapter 12.

I will show you how to use the immense power of your subconscious mind to make these common sense "habits" a regular part of your life. For years I have studied what drives top professional and Olympic athletes to succeed and in some cases overcome overwhelming obstacles, and I will share their fundamental methods for success. And in the process, I will also teach you how to master your thoughts and map your own destiny toward the desired health you truly deserve.

My goal in writing this book is to provide you with the proper tools for optimizing your health and helping you achieve the most out of life. I guarantee these 12 health habits will make a tremendous difference in your life if you truly understand and utilize what you are about to read. My only hope is that you receive as much from reading and applying these principles as I did while researching and following them myself. In fact, I have used and continue to use each one of these health principles with the greatest of success, and I know you can, too. So get ready for an exciting, eye-opening journey because the informational signposts on this trip will forever alter the course of your life. I promise!

SLIMMER, YOUNGER, STRONGER

SECTION I

BREATHE

"Whoever breathes the most air
lives the most life."

ELIZABETH BARRETT BROWNING

Chapter 1

EVERY BREATH YOU TAKE

"In all serious disease states we find a low oxygen state occurring, and low oxygen in the body tissues is a sure indicator for disease."

STEPHEN LEVINE, PH.D

What are you doing right now? Right this very instance? Are you sitting at your desk or lounging in a chair? Are you lying in bed or taking a break from your work? No matter where you are or what's going on right now, every person concentrating on this sentence has at least one thing physically in common. You are breathing air. In the time it takes for you to read this page your lungs have expanded and contracted many times. On average you breathe about 6 to 20 times per minute every hour of every day you are alive. Breathing is essential for our existence, yet most of us take it for granted.

You can live for weeks or even months without food, and you can survive several days without water, but the human organism can only live a few minutes without air. Breathing is so repetitive and so automatic you don't even think about it. Thank God for that because most of us would at one time or another forget to breathe if our brains weren't programmed to do it automatically. Why do we breathe? On the simplest level, to get oxygen into our lungs. But this natural process has more significance to it than just getting air into the body. Your breathing pattern can serve as a valuable mechanism to greatly improve your health and well-being if you understand and utilize what you are about to read.

Now that you know this chapter is about something as simple as breathing (as if you didn't know from the chapter title), you may say to yourself, "I know how to breathe" or "What's so important about breathing?"Many of the athletes and clients I have worked with felt the same way before they understood and implemented the scientific breathing principles you are about to learn. Controlling or changing your breathing pattern can greatly affect you in many ways. You may be surprised to know that just by altering your breathing, you can change your emotional state, affect your sleep cycle, improve your mental concentration, and even control your appetite. In short, your breathing pattern is more than just a process of getting air into your lungs; it can affect your health more positively (or negatively) than you could ever imagine.

THE MAGIC OF DEEP DIAPHRAGMATIC BREATHING

The special breathing pattern I am talking about is called deep, diaphragmatic breathing, and if you have ever vigorously exercised or participated in yoga or given birth, you have done some form of this type of breathing. My first encounter with this particular breathing method came when I was traveling through Europe, coaching on the World Cup circuit. I had the privilege to join my coaching counterparts from the Soviet Union to observe one of their "dryland" conditioning (weight lifting) sessions. During the intense, well-structured workout, I noticed that every athlete kept doing certain deep breathing patterns periodically throughout their exercise routine. This aroused my curiosity. As I continued to observe this process, I finally asked the host Russian coach to explain what the athletes were actually doing and why. He smiled and immediately began to praise the amazing benefits of this very interesting breathing program. He emphasized how it did wonders for the body's recuperative powers and made a noticeable improvement in the athletes' performances. I was impressed.

In all my research following that brief encounter, it is quite apparent that practicing deep, diaphragmatic breathing can indeed optimize human performance and enrich overall health. Just a few minutes a day of conscious deep, diaphragmatic breathing can help you more effectively handle negative stress, improve your immune system, sharpen your thought process, and even retard cellular aging. This concept is so simple yet so amazing that you may find it hard to believe. That is exactly why I am supporting this very unique breathing program with the latest, most credible research. Then you can decide for yourself.

Before I describe the actual deep-breathing program, I would first like to share with you what actually happens during this unusual procedure and why it is so helpful. For starters, let's look at the effects of deep, diaphragmatic breathing on the most basic cellular level. The human body is made up of approximately 60 trillion tiny little cells that perform every function necessary to sustain life. The life span of these cells can last from minutes to years, depending on a variety of environmental and genetic parameters. Simply put, the quality of your health is directly dependent on the quality of each one of your individual cells. The most crucial factors affecting their quality and life span is your body's ability to get oxygen into the cells and get waste material out. There are two major biological systems that affect how well oxygen and waste matter are transported in and away from all cells: the circulatory system and the lymphatic system.

THE CIRCULATORY SYSTEM: WHAT IS IT AND WHAT DOES IT DO?

The circulatory system is an intricate flowing structure that is comprised of a workhorse-like pump called the heart and many thousands of miles of vessels called arteries and veins. The liquid that is pumped throughout this elaborate network is called blood, and blood's primary duty is to deliver oxygen and other valuable nutrients to each and every cell. It is the amount of oxygen consistently delivered to these cells that is most crucial to their well-being. And the amount delivered is completely dependent on how efficiently your lungs take in air and extract the oxygen from it. The extracted oxygen is transported from the lungs to every cell via the circulating blood. More oxygen within the bloodstream means more available oxygen to nourish the cells.

Normal, healthy breathing usually delivers adequate oxygen in most cases. But certain environmental and biological conditions, such as stress, smoking, poor diet, sedentary lifestyle, dehydration and lack of quality sleep, are just a few examples of what can hinder oxygen delivery. People who employ deep breathing through yoga and other breathing exercises have as much as 10,000 to 20,000 more miles of capillaries than people who don't. Isn't that amazing? Having that much extra blood-circulating power can make a big difference in the nourishment of our thriving cells that ultimately makes a positive impact in our health.

The importance of how adequate levels of oxygen affect the quality and life span of our cells has been demonstrated in many scientific experiments. One such study was done by Dr. Otto Warburg, director of the Max Planck Institute for Cellular Physiology. Dr. Warburg found he could turn healthy viable cells into malignant cancerous ones simply by reducing the amount of oxygen. His study shows that cells that are insufficiently oxygenated definitely underperform their potential, and underperforming cells can lead to poorer, less than desirable health.

A follow-up study by Dr. Harry Goldblatt reported in the Journal of Experimental Medicine supported this fact. Healthy rat cells were extracted and placed into three different containers, each containing optimum levels of nutrients. Containers #1 and #2 were maintained with normal levels of oxygen, while container #3 was periodically deprived of oxygen. After one month, all the living cells in the three different containers were injected back into the healthy rats. The rats that received cells from container #1 and #2 remained healthy. However, every rat that received cells from container #3 developed cancerous tumors. "Lack of oxygen clearly plays a major role in causing cells to become cancerous," says Goldblatt. The conclusion of this experiment demonstrates how living cells depend upon adequate supplies of oxygen to remain disease free.

THE LYMPHATIC SYSTEM AND HOW IT AFFECTS YOUR HEALTH

Even if adequate oxygen is supplied, the cells cannot function at optimum levels unless resulting waste matter and other toxic material are removed efficiently from the cells. The biological system most responsible for this efficient waste removal is called the lymphatic system. This one-way system is very similar to the circulatory system. But instead of transporting nutrients to the cells via the blood, it helps carry away the waste material by way of its own fluid, called lymph. Lymph is a milky-white fluid that is contained in every space around the cells except the eyes and bones. Your body has four times more lymph fluid than blood, which demonstrates the size and importance of this powerful system.

As this lymph circulates around your body, it collects cellular waste, dead cells, unwanted foreign matter and other poisonous elements, forcing them through special filtration points called lymph nodes. These specialized nodes also produce lymphocytes, which are like armed soldiers whose main purpose is to combat this toxic material that includes invading bacteria and viruses. When you are sick, for example, you may notice that the lymph nodes around your neck swell or enlarge. This is the result of your lymph nodes working overtime to neutralize and eradicate the invading foreign material. In short, the lymphatic system is your body's mechanism for getting rid of all the unhealthy junk that builds up in and around your cells. And the freer your cellular environment is of this nasty stuff, the better it functions.

The efficiency of your lymphatic system depends on how effectively the lymph is pumped throughout your body. Simply put, the most productive cellular waste removal takes place when lymph flow is very active and forceful. Your circulatory system relies on a large powerful muscle called the heart to move blood around, but the lymphatic system must depend on other means for this pumping action. Some of the methods for assisting this lymph circulation include muscular movement, tissue massage and peristalsis of digestion. But the best, most efficient method for forcing lymph around your body is the act of deep, diaphragmatic breathing.

Several years ago, Dr. Jack Shields who is a renowned lymphologist from Santa Barbara, California, demonstrated the remarkable effects of deep, diaphragmatic breathing on the lymphatic system. By using microvideo cameras inside the body, he discovered that the act of deep, diaphragmatic breathing created a powerful lymphatic vacuum that intensified the cellular cleansing more than any other activity known. The average person has a lymph flow rate of about 125 milliliters per hour (125 ml/hour). But this experiment showed deep, diaphragmatic breathing increased the flow rate to over 1800 milliliters per hour (1800 ml/hour). In fact, the deep, diaphragmatic breathing program that I recommend in Chapter 3 increases the rate of toxic elimination by as much as 15 times the normal rate.

But how does this waste reduction affect the health and life span of your cells? One study from the Rockefeller Institute done by Dr. Alexis Carrel showed how well cells thrive in a clean environment. In this study, Dr. Carrel wanted to see how long cells would remain alive in an ideal environment, totally free of all waste matter. Cells from healthy chickens were maintained in special tubes, provided with adequate nutrients, and kept totally free of all waste and toxic material. Normal chicken cells, by the way, usually live between 10 and 12 years. After the 15-year mark, these cells were still alive and thriving. Even after 20, 25 and 30 years, these chicken cells remained alive and were still functioning at optimum levels. It was at that point that the Rockefeller Institute decided there was no need to continue this experiment any longer, since it had proven these cells could live indefinitely in a waste-free cellular environment. In humans, lymph flow is the major mechanism responsible for cleansing our cellular environment, and deep, diaphragmatic breathing is the best-known method for increasing that flow.

Current health statistics seem to back these studies. In America today, one in three women will get some form of cancerous growth sometime in their life. For men, that statistic is one in two. Pretty scary, huh? However, for people who are regularly involved in yoga or employ exercises that utilize deep, diaphragmatic breathing, the rate of getting cancer is one in seven. Degenerative diseases like cancer, arthritis, heart disease, Alzheimer's disease, chronic fatigue syndrome and premature aging have only one prime cause at the cellular level, and that is a decreased level of oxygen present. "In all serious disease states we find a low oxygen state occurring, and low oxygen in the body tissues is a sure indicator for disease," says Dr. Stephen Levine, renowned molecular biologist.

IN THE NEXT CHAPTER

After looking at this information, hopefully you can now see the tremendous importance of maintaining a healthy, oxygen-rich, waste-free cellular environment. And one of the best methods for improving the quality of your individual cells is to incorporate the daily habit of deep, diaphragmatic breathing. But deep breathing affects more than your cellular physiology, as you will soon see. Your emotional and physical well-being are directly influenced by your breathing pattern. In the next chapter you will learn how proper breathing can affect your mood, appetite, sleep and ultimately your health. So, either place a bookmark here and take a break, or go to Chapter 2, where I'll be waiting.

Chapter 2

THE BREATH OF HEALTH

"The foundation of prosperous health depends on the basic ability of getting oxygen to the cells, and deep breathing is the simplest, most fundamental method of accomplishing that."

ROBERT FULFORD, DO

BREATHING AFFECTS YOUR EMOTIONS

Not only does deep, diaphragmatic breathing affect the physiology of our cells, but it can have a dramatic effect on our emotions and stress level as well. In studying human breathing patterns it is observed that the negative emotions of fear, stress and anxiety produce more shallow-type breathing originating from the chest. On the other hand, deeper, more controlled breathing that involves the use of the diaphragm, which is a large dome-shaped muscle located in your belly, produces a more calm, relaxed emotional state. One of the best explanations of these emotional connections involves how your brain and breathing are linked neurologically. You see, the vagus nerve that runs thru the chest cavity influences the nerve receptors of the lungs and diaphragm. And the vagus nerve is directly connected to the limbic center of the brain.

The brain's limbic center influences our emotions, motivation and memory. Think about it—when you're upset you take shorter, more shallow breaths, and when you're calm and relaxed, your breaths are deeper and originate more from your diaphragm. Even though these emotional states alter your breathing pattern, the reverse can happen as well. Instead of letting your emotions control your breathing, you can manage your emotional state by purposely changing your breathing pattern. That is exactly the main concept of yoga, which uses deliberate breathing patterns to influence the mind/body connection and heighten emotional well-being. Deep breathing (like that practiced in yoga) relieves stress, slows your mind, calms you and is a valuable asset to any health program.

Deep, diaphragmatic breathing also affects the electromagnetic wavelengths in the brain. Brain wavelengths can be measured at different frequencies and are associated with various emotional states. For example, in calm, low-stress emotional states, alpha waves are predominant. A more hyped-up emotional state shows larger frequency waves, most notably delta waves. In brain wavelength experiments, deep breathing increases the formation of shorter frequency, alpha waves leading to a more relaxed mood. This could explain why your disposition becomes more serene and tranquil after several minutes of deep, diaphragmatic breathing. Furthermore, using your diaphragm to deliberately deepen your breathing pattern also affects vital health signs such as lowering blood pressure and slowing pulse rate.

On the other side of the emotional coin, negative feelings like anger and harmful stress can be directly linked to out-of-balance breathing patterns. The balance I am referring to is the cadence or rhythm of the exhale and inhale. When you become angry, the exhalation tends to be stronger and more forceful than the inhalation. And when you experience sadness the inhalations tend to be stronger. When the emotion of fear is experienced, people don't breathe much at all.

Fact is, breathing is definitely linked between the mind and our emotions. If you keep this in mind and learn to breathe more consciously, you can have greater control over your emotional state.

BREATHING AFFECTS YOUR APPETITE

Deep, diaphragmatic breathing also helps control your appetite. People who practice at least six minutes of deep breathing usually describe a feeling of satiation or stomach fullness afterwards. Although science is not really sure why this happens, many experts speculate that it's the increased oxygenated blood satisfying the cells' craving for the most important nutrient—oxygen. Also, a more dynamic lymph flow and increased activation of the diaphragm muscle contributes to feelings of stomach fullness.

There is also a psychological link between deep breathing and your desire for food. When people get stressed or worried, many tend to reach for food as a comfort or crutch. You feel down—you grab a candy bar for a pick-me-up. You're in a bad mood—you gobble a pint of ice cream to lift your spirits. It is not surprising, however, that the top reason cited for overeating is due to the psychological associations between food and emotions. By using deep, diaphragmatic breathing to ease your stress level, you more effectively disengage the emotional link between food and your appetite. So let your breathing pattern instead of food elevate your mood. Whether it's the increased blood oxygenation or emotional disassociation, correct deep breathing helps you regulate your true hunger needs.

BREATHING AFFECTS YOUR HEALTH

Poor breathing patterns or out-of-balance breathing can also contribute to ill health. Dr. Andrew Weil, a renowned alternative medical practitioner, says a disturbed breathing pattern actually creates a situation where other organs of the body are negatively affected. He goes on to say that proper breathing nourishes the brain and central nervous system and is seen to be the key to good health. In a university study, individual breathing patterns were observed in a doctor's office waiting room. It was found that 88 percent of all the people in the waiting room had disturbed breathing patterns, regardless of their physical problem. The question was posed: Does a poor breathing pattern lead to ill health, or does ill health create a poorer breathing pattern? (Or did the stress of visiting the doctor result in the disturbed breathing pattern?) Whatever the reason, the study concluded that poor breathing patterns can be linked to ill health.

A recently completed 12-year evaluation of the most successful alternative healing practices throughout our country shows just how important breathing patterns are. According to this study, the most incredible medical healer of all turns out to be an 84-year-old practicing osteopathic doctor (DO), who lives in rural Arizona. This doctor has the most incredible success rate with his patients and is described by his peers as the most effective health care clinician ever seen. What was learned most from this incredible healing doctor is how much he stresses the importance of deep breathing as an essential function of human health. Not only does he prescribe deep, diaphragmatic breathing to his patients but he does it himself daily. When asked about his health care success, he replied that the foundation of prosperous health depends on the basic ability of getting oxygen to the cells, and deep breathing is the simplest, most fundamental method of accomplishing that. Maybe that is why this successful doctor is still alive and thriving in his medical practice at the young age of 84.

When most of my elderly clients implement regular deep breathing, many of their physical ailments seem to subside or disappear altogether. One reason is the enormous amount of toxic material being released through the act of deep breathing. The human body discharges 70 percent of its toxins and waste material through breathing. Only a small percentage of this unwanted poisonous matter is discharged through sweat, defecation and urination. If your breathing is not operating at peak efficiency, you are not ridding yourself of toxins properly. But if you are deep breathing you are truly enhancing your body's ability to cleanse itself, thus promoting a healthier YOU.

HEART ATTACK AND BREATH

Deep breathing can have a very positive effect on your heart. "Coronary heart disease is due to a lack of oxygen received by the heart," says Dean Ornish, MD. A case in point is a Dutch study comparing two groups of heart attack patients. The first group was taught simple diaphragmatic breathing, while the second group was given no training in deep breathing. During a two-year period both groups were tracked. The group following a daily deep breathing program showed no signs of heart problems and did not suffer a second heart attack. However, 58 percent of the second group (those who did not follow a regular deep breathing program) had a second heart attack during the two-year period. If deep breathing can be this effective in preventing a second heart attack, just think how it can maximize your overall health and well-being.

DEEP BREATHING IMPROVES YOUR SLEEP

One of my clients, Dan, started the daily habit of deep, diaphragmatic breathing. Within a few weeks, his wife commented on how much better he was sleeping since implementing this breathing program. Before starting this regular morning and evening routine, he would toss and turn, twitch and even snore during his sleep. Dramatically, he stopped snoring after two weeks, and his twitchy body movements became less jerky. Even Dan commented on how much better and more rested he felt after adding the daily habit of deep, diaphragmatic breathing. The benefit of Dan's new breathing program is not only a better night's rest but a happier sleeping partner.

Breathing does indeed calm you, especially before sleep. It does this by slowing many of the body's metabolic processes such as blood pressure, pulse rate and brain wave activity. (Brain wave activity and successful sleep are discussed in more detail later in Chapter 7.) Deep, diaphragmic breathing also opens your air passageways and increases the capacity of your lungs. Maybe it won't completely eliminate snoring like it did in Dan's case, but it will definitely assist the function of your lungs and better prepare you for sleep.

IN THE NEXT CHAPTER

Hopefully you are now more aware of how deep, diaphragmatic breathing affects your cellular physiology and your emotional and physical health. By grasping the compelling data I have presented in the first two chapters, you are much more likely to develop the deep-breathing habit. In the next chapter you will learn the proper breathing pattern that will enable you to take advantage of its immense power and enormous healing properties. So get your body (and mind) ready for a big dose of healthy, oxygen-rich air.

Chapter 3

THE 1-3-2 BREATHING PROGRAM

"Your breathing pattern is more than just a process of getting air into your lungs; it can affect your health more positively (or negatively) than you could ever imagine."

SAM VARNER, CSCS

USING YOUR DIAPHRAGM

Chapters 1 and 2 gave you many valuable reasons for implementing the daily habit of deep diaphragmatic breathing. But what specifically is deep, diaphragmatic breathing? First of all, deep, diaphragmatic breathing is a process where the diaphragm muscle located underneath your abdominal region pulls in air to the lungs by way of the nose and windpipe. This unique, domed-shaped muscle acts like a gigantic suction device, pulling in air and expelling it with every muscular contraction. Although other muscles are involved in breathing, the diaphragm is the major one.

How do you know if you are effectively breathing with your diaphragm? A simple little method that I recommend is to place one hand over your navel and the other hand over your chest. Now slowly inhale. During your inhale try to make the hand over your navel move outward while striving to keep the other one stationary. At first, I suggest you lie on the floor, face up, to get a better feel for using your diaphragm muscle. Correct diaphragmatic breathing involves belly breathing, not chest breathing. Now, you know the basic mechanics of proper deep breathing.

DIRECTIONS FOR DEEP, DIAPHRAGMATIC BREATHING

But deep breathing involves more than just using your diaphragm. To effectively reap the maximum benefits of deep breathing, the appropriate balance of inhale to hold to exhale must be followed. Of all the programs I have studied, there are many that proved to be helpful, and all have some value if consistently followed. But the deep diaphragmatic breathing program that I recommend most is called 1-3-2 BREATHING.

Directions for the 1-3-2 BREATHING program are as follows: First, sit upright in a comfortable chair, preferably one that has a cushioned back support. Keep your back relaxed and your legs crisscrossed, with your feet as close to your groin as possible. Place your arms forward, laying them across your legs with the palms facing upward. With your eyes closed, now practice inhaling slowly through your nose by using your diaphragm. Remember, be a belly breather, not a chest breather.

Take as long as possible to inhale. For most people, that's between 6 to 8 seconds. Once your lungs are full, hold your breathe for 3 times as long as it took you to inhale. Now slowly release through your mouth the held air. Try to exhale for twice as long as your inhale count was. The inhale and exhale should be done quietly without forcing the air.

With your eyes shut, picture pleasant thoughts and tranquil places, especially during the exhale portion. The exhale phase is the most beneficial to the mind and body because this is where the healthy "feel-good" hormones called endorphins are released. It is also where you usually experience a more soothing sensation. (Maybe that's why you feel relief after long sighs.) In other words, the exhale provides the most relaxation.

Again your breathing ratios of inhale-to-hold-to-exhale should be 1-to-3-to-2—hence the name 1-3-2 BREATHING. For example, if it takes you a 6-count to inhale, then hold your filled lungs for an 18-count (6 times 3) and exhale through your mouth for a 12-count (6 times 2). Repeat this breathing cycle for a total of ten times in the morning and ten times in the evening. It will take you about four to six minutes to complete each session.

GETTING THE MOST OUT OF 1-3-2

And what makes this breathing method work? During the inhale portion, the diaphragm pulls in air through your nose and fills your lungs. By holding the air in your lungs, the blood oxygen level (blood oxygenation) increases, which means more valuable oxygen is delivered to your cells. Once you release the stored air from your lungs by way of your mouth, the thoracic duct of your lymphatic system opens immediately, thus flushing lymph fluid throughout your body at a more forceful rate. You may recall from an earlier discussion how increased lymph flow helps to improve cellular waste removal and enhances your immune system. This is the cornerstone of the 1-3-2 breathing program.

Remember, inhale, hold, and exhale for a count ratio of 1 to 3 to 2. For added benefit, visualize pleasant and relaxing pictures in your mind while performing this daily breathing program. (I will discuss in more detail the mental aspects of visualization in Chapter 11.) I recommend that you do this special breathing program in the morning and evening for optimum benefits. However, you may, for that matter, do deep, diaphragmatic breathing as many times during the day as you want.

Do a few 1-3-2 BREATHING cycles while watching TV or sitting at a stoplight or waiting in line. In fact you can do it right now; it's like taking an oxygen cocktail. I cannot stress enough the importance of implementing regular, daily deep breathing, especially the 1-3-2 deep, diaphragmatic breathing program. Your long-term health benefits will be immeasurable. Please try this breathing program for 30 days, and I guarantee you will notice a difference—a major difference!

SUMMARY

Why is deep, diaphramic breathing so important?

1. Helps controls appetite.
2. Improves the quality of your sleep.
3. Improves the function of living cells by increasing the flow of oxygen.
4. Promotes a healthier cellular environment by increasing lymph flow as much as 15 times the normal rate, which allows for better removal of cellular waste. (In other words, it cleanses the cells.)
5. Elevates endorphin hormones that promote an overall sense of euphoria and well-being. (It makes you feel good.)
6. Promotes positive changes in brain electromagnetic wavelength activity, creating a more calm and relaxed emotional state of mind.
7. Reduces negative stress and improves your mood.

Following the recommended deep, diaphragmatic breathing in Health Habit 12 can promote a more healthy mind and body in less than 12 minutes a day. The human being has within it a remarkable power to fight disease, heal itself, and achieve optimum health. The act of deep, diaphragmatic breathing is one of nature's most valuable tools in helping you accomplish that.

HEALTH HABIT 12:

Practice deep, diaphragmatic breathing at least ten minutes in the morning and ten minutes in the evening. Inhale, hold, and exhale your breath for a cadence of 1 to 3 to 2. Repeat this 1-3-2 breathing cycle for a total of 10 times in the morning and 10 times in the evening. For example, if it takes you a 6-count to inhale, then hold your filled lungs for an 18-count (6 times 3) and exhale through your mouth for a 12-count (6 times 2).

SECTION II

EAT

"Let thy food be thy medicine and thy medicine be thy food."

HIPPOCRATES

Chapter 4

THINK BEFORE YOU DRINK

"If there were a fountain of youth, it would flow with water—cool, sparkling and life sustaining."
WINIFRED CONKLING

Second to the air we breathe, the human body needs water the most. Water is the most valuable liquid on earth, and not one living creature could exist without it. In fact, most people can survive only 5 to 10 days without this precious element. But what makes water so special? Why does the human body require water? How much water does the body actually need? And are there any health benefits to drinking lots of waters?

To understand the need for water, let us first look at how it is used in the body. As discussed in Section I, the health of the body is dependent on the health of the individual cells that make it up. Water is present in and around every living cell and is involved in every cellular activity that takes place. From digestion to perspiration, from the flow of blood to the removal of waste, water affects every activity. Each cell contains countless chemicals, minerals, vitamins, and other nutrients that all function best when they are bathed in the right amount of water-containing fluid.

THE MANY ROLES OF WATER

Water has many roles in the body. It acts as a coolant, lubricating agent, transport vehicle, solvent and detoxifier, to name a few. The blood that is pulsing around in your veins right now is made up of over 85 percent water. Its thickness or viscosity is in part due to the amount of water you consume. Seventy-five percent of your brain and 70 percent of your muscles are made up of water. Water helps regulate your body temperature much like the water in a car radiator. The underconsumption of water can greatly affect your body's ability to maintain an ideal body temperature, especially in hot or dry climates.

Water helps cushion the joints and protects all the vital organs and tissues. Water helps dissolve and eliminate waste material and by-products that build up from cellular metabolism. Water is the key element involved in the lymphatic system, which, if you recall from Chapter 1, is the primary system in charge of cellular cleansing. In fact, your lymph fluid is made up mostly of water, which affects the quality of your immune system. This means your disease-fighting and toxic neutralization capabilities are directly dependent on adequate water intake. This a must for optimum health!

Water is also the best-known solvent. Being a solvent means it dissolves or hydrolyzes material into smaller, more usable parts. Food, for example, is broken down into its smaller chemical elements with the help of water. The act of digestion is much more efficient if your body is well hydrated. Water also helps breakdown toxic chemical residue that may be present in many of the foods you consume. Optimum water consumption thus facilitates a more rapid excretion of these unwanted materials. Besides cellular waste and food toxins, there are also many other chemical pollutants that enter your body from various environmental sources, which water helps to neutralize and discard.

Nowadays people are exposed to modern-day toxic chemicals such as pesticides, heavy metals, residue from pharmaceutical drugs and many illegal drugs that adversely affect our long-term health. The American diet of saturated fats, sugars, caffeine, alcohol and other undesirable chemicals also puts a great strain on our living tissues. Underconsumption of water in an already junk-filled environment like the typical American diet greatly represses the body's ability to heal itself. In spite of all the ill effects of poor eating habits and an ever-increasing polluted environment, the proper consumption of water can make a big difference by negating some of these adverse effects.

Water is also the best-known human cleansing agent. An increase in water intake can help detoxify the body from many of the negative chemical buildups, thereby providing a rejuvenation effect for all its cells. This rejuvenation effect improves the organisms' ability to fight disease and illness. Even bad nutrition can be offset somewhat by increased water intake. A great example of the power of water as a cleansing agent can be seen in the remarkable health benefits of the juice fast. The success of many juice fast programs is primarily due to the additional intake of nutrient-rich fruit and vegetable juice that contains over 95 percent pure, natural water. The ability to assist the body's removal of the poisonous, unwanted chemical and cellular by-products is directly affected by the amount of water you consume.

ARE YOU REALLY GETTING ENOUGH WATER?

Statistics show 50 percent of Americans think they are getting enough water on a regular basis. Since the adequate consumption of water is so crucial to the quality of human health, it would reason that abundant water intake would prevail in our society. However, a study conducted by the Nutrition Information Center at the New York Hospital Cornell Medical Center found most Americans are only getting about one third of the water they need. In the same survey of 3,003

Americans, only 21 percent of the respondents said they drink the recommended eight or more glasses of water a day, while 35 percent drink fewer than 3 glasses a day. The average daily intake of water, according to this medical survey, is only 4.6 glasses a day, far below what the body actually needs for optimum health.

But the real problem is not only the lack of daily water intake but the amount of water-depleting beverages that are consumed. Water-depleting beverages act as a diuretic, causing the body to lose excess water through urination. Alcoholic and caffeinated beverages such as coffee, soda pop, liquor, beer and wine are the most common ones that siphon water from our tissues and rapidly create cellular dehydration. "The vast majority of people aren't drinking enough water to begin with," says Barbara Levine, spokesperson for the Cornell Medical Center, "and to make matters worse, many don't realize that beverages containing alcohol and caffeine actually rob the body of water." Even if you intentionally drink eight glasses of water during the day, but you consume a couple of cups of coffee in the morning, a couple of diet sodas during the day and a glass of wine in the evening, you only receive the net effectiveness of three glasses of water. That's right! The coffee, soda and alcohol just canceled out most of your diligent water intake. So beware of the negative effects of water-depleting beverages, and try to consume enough water to offset their intake. Better yet, for optimum health give up the water-depleting beverages altogether. Your cells will love you.

But just how much water is really needed? Let's first look at how much water your body actually uses. The natural outflow of water from your body is around 64 to 80 ounces a day. That's 8 to 10 glasses. Water is lost through urination, breathing (vapor loss), perspiration and even bowel movements. In fact, the average person produces around two and a half pints of urine a day and loses over 2 cups of water vapor just through breathing. So the minimum amount of water just to replace the normal fluid loss would need to be 8 to 10 glasses a day, and that amount is increased if you are exercising, pregnant, breast-feeding, live in a dry environment or are sick. Even flying in a commercial airliner can deplete your water stores rapidly due to the incredibly dry cabin environment. However, for optimum health, just consuming the minimum amount your body loses is simply not enough.

HEALTH CONSEQUENCES OF ADEQUATE AND INADEQUATE WATER INTAKE

If you are not getting at least eight glasses of water a day, your cells aren't getting enough of what they need. You're just asking for trouble! The most common side effect of not consuming enough water is fatigue or reduced energy levels. Continued inadequate water intake can lead to headache, weakness, dizziness and lack of concentration. However, the long-term effects of insufficient hydration will affect your ability to fight off infection and disease. And it will definitely show up in how you look.

In terms of appearance, your skin tone is a very important indicator of ample water intake. When enough water is present, the skin has more elasticity and better color, and it ages much more slowly. A good example of this is seen in singer and entertainer, Tina Turner. Here is a very beautiful lady who definitely looks 20 years younger than she really is, especially her youthful skin. When an interviewer asked her what her secret was to looking young and being so energetic, she replied that it was due in part to drinking an enormous amount of water daily.

Furthermore, there are countless fashion models who indicate they drink at least eight glasses of water a day to promote youthful-looking skin and enrich their natural beauty. It's true. And almost every beauty book or cosmetic magazine on the subject will tell you to do the same. So if you want to preserve your youthful look, enhance your skin complexion, and maintain plenty of energy, consume lots of water and I mean lots of it.

HOW MUCH WATER SHOULD I DRINK?

Studies show the amount of water consumed each day should be between 2 and 3 percent of one's body weight. So for someone with a body weight of 150 pounds, daily consumption of water should be around 72 ounces (3 percent x 150 x 16 oz = 72 oz). That's nine cups (8-ounce size) of water per day for an average weight individual. Sound like a lot? Not really when you consider the awesome advantages ample water intake delivers.

So, what's the best way to accomplish my daily water intake? Drinking filtered water is the most common method of achieving your suggested intake. Distilled water is also okay but not as beneficial because the distillation process removes many of the essential trace elements needed by your body. But let's not split hairs here. The idea is to consume lots of pure water throughout the day. I recommend that you drink 10 or more glasses or at least 80 ounces of water per day, minimum. And, no, don't count the liquid in diet sodas, tea and milk. Remember to subtract alcoholic and caffeinated beverages, as they increase water loss. What I mean is drink pure water, as pure as you can get it.

The act of drinking water needs to be a conscious effort. You cannot wait for the thirst mechanism to signal water consumption. "The thirst mechanism isn't very sensitive, and it doesn't kick in until dehydration becomes serious," says dehydration expert David D. Schnakenberg, Ph.D., executive officer of the American Society of Clinical Nutrition. Usually by the time you feel the thirst urge, your body is already in a water deficit. You see, human beings are the only animal whose true thirst mechanism is not in sync with the need for water. Maybe it's the constant chemical and environmental abuse our living tissues endure or the common practice of overindulging in water-depleting fluids that creates this out-of-sync water alarm. Whatever the reason, don't wait for the thirst urge to strike; consciously make an effort to drink this most valuable liquid throughout the day, every day!

WHEN TO DRINK

For some people who have a tough time consuming their water quota, I suggest this easy method for remembering. Simply drink 12 to 24 ounces of water upon arising every morning (see Health Habit 10) and 10 to 12 ounces of water before every meal and snack (see Health Habit 11). Also, drink a glass of water before and after each physical workout. This will ensure enough water intake without having to cart around a water bottle all day long. Don't get me wrong. It's okay to carry around your filtered water supply if that helps you consume your recommended allotment. But it's probably more convenient to satisfy your water need if you develop the daily habit of intentionally drinking water when you wake up, before each meal, and after each workout.

Besides, drinking water before meals has been proven to reduce food consumption and help control appetite. The thirst signal sent from the hypothalamus is often confused with hunger, resulting in eating when you're not really hungry—just thirsty. So, by maintaining a well-hydrated state, you minimize this thirst/hunger confusion, thus cutting down on your food intake.

Also, too many people drink beverages with their meals, and research shows that the more you drink with your meals, the less you chew your food. And the less you chew your food, the faster you eat. And the faster you eat, the more food your stomach receives before it signals the brain to stop eating. The result is you usually eat too much. So for best results, drink water before your meals and not during your meals (and chew your food more thoroughly as well). No matter what motivates you, just remember to drink lots of pure water immediately after arising and before every meal and workout. This will more than guarantee satisfactory water intake.

WARM WATER AND LEMON JUICE

Consuming 12 to 24 ounces of warm water with fresh lemon juice first thing in the morning is one of the healthiest ways to cleanse your system and detoxify your cells. The fresh lemon juice aids in the additional cleansing and "detox" of the liver and colon, while providing vital phytonutrients and beneficial natural enzymes. This particular citrus juice contains very potent antiviral and antibacterial agents that help ward off colds and other minor illnesses. Also research suggests that the scent of fresh lemon has an energizing effect as well. Make sure the lemon is fresh, not bottled. Not only does this particular citrus juice help nourish some of your internal organs, it also adds a pleasant flavor to the warm water. Try it, you might actually enjoy your "lemon-water time" in the mornings. I do!

Warm or hot water as opposed to cold seems to soothe the body, especially in the morning. A water temperature between 90 and 100 degrees (Fahrenheit) works best because it allows for more optimum absorption and is less stressful to your digestive system. Even though cold water doesn't pose any serious harm, warm water is more soothing and acceptable at this time of day. I have this instead of coffee; it's a whole lot healthier and has no side effects.

Is it possible to drink too much water? The answer for healthy individuals is an emphatic NO! As a matter of fact, your kidneys thrive on excess water. That's their job. Abundant water intake helps your kidneys perform more effectively and at a higher level of efficiency. Besides, they need the work. Sometimes I'm asked if drinking too much water during your meals will interfere with the digestive enzymes and nutrient absorption. My reply is absolutely not. No matter how much water you consume, your intestinal tract will still absorb the available nutrients with no negative effects on the digestive or enzymatic process. The fiber you eat also loves the extra water. It is water that this fiber binds with to facilitate a better intestinal cleansing as it exits the body. So drink, drink, drink that magical liquid.

THE BEST WATER SOURCE

However, not all the water that enters your system comes from what you drink. In fact, the very best source of this natural mineral-laced liquid comes from water-rich foods. That's right! Believe it or not, fresh vegetables, sprouts and fruits contain over 85 percent naturally filtered fluid and are the best possible sources of water. Not only is the water in these raw, edible plants naturally purified, it also contains essential vitamins, minerals and easily absorbable trace elements. So, you not only want to drink lots of water throughout the day, you also need to eat plenty of fresh vegetables and fruits for their water content value as well.

Sadly enough, it is a fact that most people do not consume enough water or get enough natural liquid through healthy eating. Developing the daily habit of drinking lots of water and eliminating water-depleting beverages will help ensure better health and vitality. The most motivating reasons for consciously developing the water-drinking habit is how you look and feel. Your energy level will noticeably improve, and your skin tone and complexion will especially show the benefits of abundant water intake. Just think about all those trillions of cells within your body that will thrive when you bathe them with lots of healthy, pure, natural water. Your health does indeed depend on how much water you drink. So think before you drink.

HEALTH HABIT 11:

Drink a full glass (10 to 12 ounces) of filtered water before every meal and snack, and before and after all exercise.

HEALTH HABIT 10:

Drink approximately 12 to 24 ounces of warm water with fresh lemon juice from half a lemon upon arising every morning.

Chapter 5

IN SEARCH OF FOOD

"Food has a more powerful impact on your body and your health than any drug your doctor could ever prescribe."

BARRY SEARS, PHD

After retiring as a conditioning coach, I entered the business of personal fitness training, where I continued to help others improve their physical health and well-being. One important aspect of getting people into tip-top shape is to instruct them on sound nutrition and encourage them to follow through with good eating habits. With a BS degree in food science-nutrition and biology, I felt very competent in training and assisting my clients in the health field, especially nutrition.

However, the one thing that really discouraged me in assisting some of my overweight clients was the few who didn't reach their fat-loss goals. Now don't misunderstand me; I was very pleased with the successes of most of my clients; but the perfectionist in me could not accept these few failures. When a client would not successfully complete a fat-loss goal but claimed to follow the nutritional and exercise guidelines set forth, I couldn't understand it. In situations like this, I simply thought these particular clients just didn't follow the suggested program. After all, the dietary plan I recommended was the accepted low-fat, high-complex-carbohydrate nutritional approach. At least that is the current conventional wisdom of most nutritionists and doctors.

However, I did notice that the clients who made the most progress in attaining a leaner, healthier body did the most exercise. In fact, the average clients who succeeded in their fat-loss goals did over an hour of exercise a day. The biggest problem here is that most people don't have that much time to devote to formal exercise. Could there be a better way? Was there something I was missing in the health and weight loss arena?

With this burning question, I decided to delve deeper into the nutrition field. Even though it had been over twenty years since my college studies, I started reading and examining all the latest material on cellular physiology, biochemistry and almost every creditable nutrition publication I could find. I even looked at other areas that might shed light on how the human body was designed to eat. Books on anthropology, disease, cultural eating habits and even the Holy Bible were involved in my investigation.

I began to notice some very interesting correlations between the foods we eat and the various hormones our body secretes. It seems the human body hormonally responds quite differently to each of the three major food components. The three components I am referring to are carbohydrates, fats and proteins, otherwise known as macronutrients. What I found most interesting in all my nutritional research was the emergence of a definite relationship between carbohydrate intake and being overweight. That's right. My research was pointing toward excessive carbohydrate consumption as a major contributor to obesity, even more so than fat intake. This really blew me away, since I had been recommending a high-complex-carbohydrate, low-fat diet to my clients and athletes for so many years. But how much does this carbohydrate intake influence fat storage?

To hopefully answer this question, I decided to investigate the sport of bodybuilding. The reason for looking at this highly competitive sport is that these types of athletes are extremely successful in achieving very low body fat levels. Most top female bodybuilders will attain body fat levels as low as 5 percent, while their male counterparts will achieve even lower levels. I wondered what kind of diet these athletes followed to reach such low levels of body fat.

As it turns out, in order to accomplish this lean and muscular physique, bodybuilders lower their intake of carbohydrates, while maintaining a moderate protein intake. In fact, most professional bodybuilders will cut their carbohydrate intake to extremely low levels just days before competition. This seemingly unhealthy practice has been done for years in the sport of bodybuilding with great success. Keep in mind, however, that these dedicated athletes spend an enormous amount of time exercising to look the way they do. Nevertheless, any bodybuilder will tell you that diet is the key to reducing body fat levels. And surprisingly the key to a fat-reducing diet is the amount of carbohydrates consumed.

But how important is this carbohydrate restriction? And what carbohydrates are restricted to help these bodybuilders become the leanest? In my research to answer these questions, I began to observe a deeper, more alarming connection between the foods we eat and the disease states prevalent in our society. My investigation kept pointing toward a link between our body's hormonal response to certain food types and our susceptibility to illness. Maybe this hormonal thing has as much to do with our overall health as it does with the incidence of obesity. Well, I got the idea to look at our nation's eating habits to see if I could draw any correlations to our health as a whole. Maybe this would lead somewhere.

DOES FOOD AFFECT OUR HEALTH?

One such national report really caught my eye. The Surgeon General's Report on Nutrition and Health stated, "What we eat may affect our risk for several of the leading causes of death for Americans, notably the degenerative disease such as: heart disease, diabetes and some types of cancer. All together, these disorders now account for more than two thirds of the deaths in the United States."This year twice as many people in this country will die as a result of cardiovascular disease and diabetes than all Americans that died in World War I, World War II, the Korean and the Vietnam Wars combined. Every person reading this knows someone who has been or is currently afflicted with heart disease, diabetes or cancer.

Cancer is a growing scourge that continues to afflict our nation. One in four American deaths this year will be the result of cancer. One in three women and one in two men will get some form of cancer within their lifetime. There are 1,400,000 new cancer cases reported each year, and with a death rate of 35 percent, nearly 500,000 people will die as a result. However, the latest research shows that more than 70 percent of all cancer is preventable and 40 percent is directly related to the foods we eat. That's right, your day-to-day lifestyle choices can drastically affect your chances of contracting this horrible disease.

Obesity is another increasing problem in our society that is definitely diet related. One in three people in the United States is obese. Nearly 60 percent of Americans are overweight, with some reports showing up to 65 percent being overweight. Even one in five children is overweight. However, statistics show that people are consuming less fat today than they did 10 years ago. Since 1970, dietary fat intake has actually decreased 16 percent. A survey sampling shows people nowadays are more health conscious than ever before, especially when it comes to their eating habits.

With more nutritional awareness and the availability of lower-fat foods, you would think that Americans would show dramatic signs of improved health. Current facts, however, do not bear this out. In reality, the opposite is occurring. Believe it or not, obesity is continuing to rise at an alarming rate. This affliction has risen in the last decade by a whopping 25%. Also, the occurrences of heart disease, diabetes and hypertension have increased as well. Why is that? Do these statistics really make sense? If people are now more cognizant of what to eat and are consuming less dietary fat, then why the increase in these food-related diseases?

WHAT DID OUR ANCESTORS EAT?

Maybe the answers to my questions can be found in our past. After all, if you can't learn from your past, you are destined to repeat it. In 1982, Claire Cassidy, PhD, from the University of Maryland and the Smithsonian Institute, presented her findings on studies of two different cultures from the same geographical area. Almost every environmental aspect was identical including climate and gene pool. The two major differences were the time they lived and the food they ate.

One group, the hunters, lived around 3000 B.C. and consumed mostly fish, mussels, deer and wild turkey, along with some wild plants. They were called the Indian Knolls group, and their diet would be classified as high-protein. The second group, the farmers, ate mostly farmed items such as corn, beans, grains and very little wild game. They were called the Hardin Village group and ate mainly an agricultural diet high in complex carbohydrates.

By studying the skeletal remains, Dr. Cassidy was able to analyze and compare the overall health of both cultures. Even though both cultures were genetically alike, some major difference were noted. The farmers had a life expectancy much lower than that of the hunters.

Evidence of infection was 13 times more prevalent in the farmers than the hunters. Tooth decay was much more widespread in the farmers and almost nonexistent in the hunters. To quote Dr. Cassidy, "The agricultural Hardin Villagers (farmers) were clearly less healthy than the Indian Knollers (hunters), who lived by hunting and gathering." She goes on to say, "The health data provides convincing evidence that the diet of the agriculturists was the inferior of the two. The archaeological dietary data support this conclusion."

Other anthropological studies bear this out. Prior to 8,000 years ago, man's diet consisted mainly of meat, nuts, seeds and berries. After that time, the most notable dietary changes took place with the agricultural revolution, and that is where archaeologists noticed definite changes in the structure and health of our ancestors. The condition of our ancestral hunters before the agricultural period showed a taller, stronger bone structure with fewer health problems compared to the more recent (within the last 8,000 years) agricultural period farmers, who showed higher rates of disease, malnutrition and tooth decay. The main difference in the diets of the two periods in question is the ratio of protein to carbohydrates to fats. And the higher the ratio of carbohydrates, the a higher the incidence of health problems. You would think it would be the higher-fat ratio that would cause the health problems. But none of these anthropological studies demonstrated a fat-to-disease link. This would tend to corroborate how important our carbohydrate intake is to our overall health.

HORMONES AND FOOD

In further research, I found the nutrition field was turned upside down in 1982 with a study involving the glycemic index. The glycemic index is the measure of how much a given food will raise your blood sugar level upon entering the blood-stream. What this study demonstrated is that all foods are not absorbed equally in the body. When you ingest food, it is broken down into smaller elements by digestion and then absorbed into the bloodstream. The carbohydrates in your food are broken down into simple sugars, with glucose being the simplest.

When these sugars are absorbed into the bloodstream at faster than acceptable rates, your blood sugars rise. This rapid rise in your blood sugar level results in the oversecretion of a hormone called insulin. Insulin is a very powerful master hormone secreted by the pancreas in an effort to help stabilize high blood sugar levels. If your blood sugar level becomes too low, then the insulin counterpart hormone called glucagon is secreted. Actually, your bloodstream has both hormones flowing around all the time. But it's the types of ingested food and how much you eat that creates the change in the blood levels of these very powerful hormones.

Your brain needs this sugar in your blood for fuel. In fact, it's the only organ of the body that uses glucose entirely as its energy supply. The brain likes the supply of blood sugar (glucose) to be balanced and consistent. This organ hates high levels of blood sugars as well as low levels. Fluctuation of blood sugar levels affects most noticeably your mood. However, extreme fluctuations can eventually lead to some very serious health problems, as you will soon learn. In short, insulin and glucagon are responsible for the balancing act of your blood sugars.

A big problem with a rapid increase in blood sugar levels is that your pancreas overcompensates by secreting too much insulin. And too much insulin reduces the blood sugar levels too rapidly. One noticeable effect of this high/low blood sugar ride is the drastic emotional state changes seen in people with fluctuating blood sugars. A prime example is a state of hyperactivity immediately after a sugary meal that is usually followed by a state of lethargy or tiredness. This is somewhat of an oversimplification of the process, but the point is that too much sugar entering the bloodstream affects how much insulin is secreted. And elevated blood insulin levels affect not only your mood but many other instrumental functions of the body as well. Please keep this in mind.

The brain and your mood are not the only elements affected by the rapid rise and fall of blood sugar levels. In fact, every cell in your body is greatly affected by this roller-coaster ride. When insulin is secreted to stabilize higher levels of blood sugar, where does this extra sugar go? Well, some sugar is stored in the muscle tissue for fueling muscular contractions. But a large part of this excess sugar is stored in the adipose tissue as fat. You see, insulin's primary duty is to regulate blood sugar levels by allocating how much sugar goes into your fat cells for storage and muscle tissue for energy. And too much sugar stimulating too much insulin translates into more fat stored.

What does the glycemic index have to do with all this? Well, prior to its study, science had generalized that simple sugars eaten in excess would spike blood sugar levels, while complex carbohydrates would not. In other words, simple sugars such as candy and sweets were made out to be the bad guys, and complex carbohydrates like grains and pastas were the good guys. The big revelation from the glycemic index study shows that not all complex carbohydrate foods enter the bloodstream at such a slow, steady pace, as was previously thought.

In fact, the highest glycemic-rated foods, which are foods that raise blood sugars the fastest, are processed carbohydrate foods like white breads, plain pasta, chips and rice cakes. What this means is that foods like rice cakes and most breads, for example, may contribute to body fat storage even more than candy. Shocking, huh? And that's why the nutrition field was thrown on its ear, so to speak, back in 1982. Of course, there are other factors that affect the sugar absorption rate, such as fiber, fat and protein content. But nevertheless, the carbohydrates in the foods you eat play a major role in blood sugar levels and insulin production.

The insulin response to food is much more sophisticated and complicated than I have described here. But I've tried to make it simple enough so that everyone can see how our bodies hormonally respond to the foods we eat. The bottom line is that too many processed carbohydrate-rich foods stimulate the body to secrete too much insulin. And excess insulin is the major culprit in fat storage. (Excess calories also stimulate too much insulin.) In fact, another name for insulin is the fat-storing hormone. But insulin is much more than a blood sugar regulator and a fat-storing hormone. So, what else does insulin do and how does it affect you?

WHAT DOES INSULIN DO?

Until just recently, controlling blood sugar levels was thought to be insulin's only important role. But new scientific research sheds an entirely different light by showing that this master hormone affects other important cellular activities as well. For example, higher than normal blood insulin levels promote an increase in cholesterol production. Elevated insulin levels increase the smooth muscle tissue within the artery walls. And high blood insulin levels inhibit the kidneys from removing excess water and sodium. So, what do these biological events have to do with good health? Well, let's examine each one and see.

Elevated levels of cholesterol are linked to cardiovascular disease. In fact, the average cholesterol reading of a heart attack victim is 267 (ml/dl). But what causes this high level of cholesterol? For the most part, diet is still maintained by many as the contributor to high cholesterol. However, less than 20 percent of all the cholesterol in your body comes from your diet. Eighty-percent of this waxy, gooey substance is produced mainly by your very own liver. That's right. Your liver makes most of it. But what causes the liver to over-secrete such undesirable levels of cholesterol. Insulin! Surprised?

Continued oversecretion of insulin causes the liver to make excess cholesterol, which finds its way into your bloodstream. In fact, excessive insulin levels have more of an effect on your blood cholesterol reading than the fat and cholesterol in your diet. Interesting, huh? So, if you want to lower your blood cholesterol, reduce the amount of insulin in your blood. And how do you reduce the amount of blood insulin? Think about it for a moment...

Another result of excess insulin is the increase in smooth muscle tissue within the artery walls. More muscle tissue within the artery walls decreases the diameter of blood flow. This narrowing of the passageway generates a greater blood-flow pressure that contributes to hypertension. In short, high blood pressure can now be scientifically and medically linked to elevated insulin levels. Most medical professionals agree that the food you eat is a major contributor to hypertension and lay most the blame on salt intake. I agree that the food you eat affects your blood pressure, but it's not so much the salt intake as it is the insulin-promoting foods you eat.

Not only does excess insulin contribute to elevated cholesterol and high blood pressure, but it affects the ability of your kidneys to remove excess sodium and other salts from your tissue. This disruption causes the body to retain water, thus promoting swelling and edema. So, it is not so much the extra salt you ingest, it's the excessive insulin level that results in the kidney's inability to remove it. In fact, a recent study just released confirms that salt intake affects blood pressure and edema much less than previously thought. It's the insulin, people!

Chronically high levels of insulin contribute to heart disease. As far back as the early 1960s this was proven in animal experiments. Dr. Anatolio Cruz demonstrated this in an experiment where he injected insulin into the leg arteries of dogs every day for seven months. He also used a control group where he injected a saline solution instead. At the end of the experiment, the arteries injected with the saline solution were examined and found to be normal. However, the arteries injected with insulin were almost completely clogged with cholesterol and fatty material. Also the inner artery lining had become much thicker compared to the control group. This shows the dramatic effects of excessive insulin on living animals for only a short period. Just think what happens to humans whose cells are exposed to excessive insulin during a lifetime. As a matter of fact, medical observers are finding higher than normal insulin levels in almost every human disease state. And again, what contributes to elevated insulin levels? THINK!

Most of the earth-shattering revelations about hormone nutrition, disease, and our health have come within the last five years. However, it was one of the earlier investigations done by Dr. Robert Atkins that really initiated the paradigm shift in the nutritional information that you are now seeing. He combined research from Dr. Garfield Duncan of the University of Pennsylvania and two English researchers, Professor Kekwick and Dr. Pawan, to devise some very revolutionary nutritional guidelines. He concluded that lowering dietary carbohydrates results in lowering insulin levels, which is very significant for improving health and vitality and most directly related to effective fat loss.

His dietary claims were so controversial and so contradictory to mainstream nutrition when they were first presented in the late 1960s that he was called before a Senate subcommittee and lambasted for his antithetic viewpoints. Even though his earlier research and dietary recommendations were not widely accepted, his patients greatly benefitted from his nutritional convictions. However, in the last five years more conclusive medical and nutritional research seems to be supporting the premise that diet and elevated insulin levels are directly related to our overall health.

In most cases, diseases like heart disease, cancer, hypertension, diabetes, and obesity are related to what we eat. It is suggested by some of the top nutritional researchers that these diseases, especially obesity, are not diseases in and of themselves but only symptoms of a greater dilemma in our society. Too much insulin! Could this excessive insulin be the contributing factor to some of our country's major diseases? It certainly appears so, but I still need more proof.

A NEW HORMONE?

To further support the relationship between the foods we eat and the health we experience, a new, more powerful class of hormones have come to the forefront within the last 25 years. These very unique hormones are called eicosonoids, and their findings are already starting to change the way science views human health. In fact, the initial discovery was so remarkable that the 1982 Nobel Prize for Physiology and Medicine was awarded to three scientists, Sune Bergstrom, Bengt Samuelsson, and John Vane, for their extensive research in this area.

What's so incredible about eicosonoids is that they control almost every function in the human body on a cellular level. They are produced within the cells and are not specific to any special gland like other known hormones. Unlike any other hormone, they are not found in the bloodstream, and they have a very short life span, which makes them very difficult to measure and observe.

There are two classes of eicosonoids, called series I and series II. Both series of hormones affect important bodily functions such as blood pressure, immune response, inflammatory reaction, pain/fever cycles, sleep/wake cycles, artery constriction and dilation, airway constriction and dilation, cellular growth, platelet formation, and many others. The difference between series I and series II eicosonoids is that each has a countering effect. In simpler terms, series I has the most positive effects on your health, and series II has the most negative. Hence, the most common names assigned to these special hormones are "good" eicosonoids, referring to series I, and "bad" eicosonoids, referring to series II. With this discovery, and with better detection of eicosonoids, health and well-being can now be scientifically defined by the ratio of good eicosonoids to bad ones. In other words, if you desire optimum health, then good eicosonoid production must be maintained and bad eicosonoid production should be minimized.

HOW CAN GOOD EICOSONOIDS BE MAINTAINED?

There are several methods for maintaining series I eicosonoids in your system. The most effective way to support the optimum level of good eicosonoid hormones is by maintaining a proper insulin-glucagon balance. Does this sound familiar? And the most effective way of maintaining a proper insulin-glucagon hormonal balance is by eating a diet containing the proper ratio of protein to carbohydrates to fats. In other words, a diet containing low-processed carbohydrates, adequate protein and healthy fats is the best method for maintaining good eicosonoid levels.

Another important method for maintaining good eicosonoid levels is with a diet containing adequate amounts of an essential fatty acid called linoleic acid. Before you rush out to ransack General Nutrition Center for linoleic acid supplements, note the best sources of this valuable nutrient can be found right in the foods you eat. A diet rich in fibrous vegetables, raw nuts and seeds all contain this essential nutrient in ample amounts. But just getting linoleic acid into your diet is not enough. Absorption is the key. You could have an abundant amount of this nutrient circulating around your system, but it is the absorption of this valuable nutrient that's essential for proper utilization.

Aging, stress, and diet all affect the absorption of linoleic acid. Aging is inevitable, but the health habits described in this book will greatly improve your cells'resistance to age. Stress is also present in our lives, but how you deal with it is the biggest key. Your eating habits also play a major role in proper linoleic acid absorption. Ironically, the same diet that aids linoleic acid absorption is the same diet that supports good eicosonoid production.

There are six fundamental dietary guidelines for achieving optimum levels of good eicosonoids within your cells:

1. Eat a low-processed carbohydrate diet by reducing the amount of white flour and refined sugar products such as breads, pastries, candy, chips and soda pop.
2. Add healthy oils and fats to your diets, such as raw nuts, seeds and monounsaturated oils such as olive oil. Olive oil is one of the best oils for cooking and use in salad dressings.
3. Eat adequate amounts of protein, which assures proper eicosonoid production. A diet containing at least 30 percent protein is recommended.
4. Limit trans-fatty acid products such as margarine and hard fats. These types of foods elevate bad eicosonoids.
5. Increase the consumption of foods containing EPA oil (eicosapentaenoic acid), which are contained in the omega-3 fish oils. Cold-water fish such as salmon, herring and mackerel should be eaten at least three to six times a week. EPA oil is a great stimulator of good eicosonoids.
6. Reduce the fat intake from certain foods such as red meats, organ meats and egg yolks. These fats contain a substance called arachidonic acid that may elevate bad eicosonoids in some individuals. Not everyone is sensitive to this acid, but as a precaution, I recommend trimming off visible fat from red meats, avoiding organ meats, and using egg whites or Egg Beaters instead of whole eggs. Also, grilling meats is more beneficial than frying in terms of arachidonic acids.

In a typical low-fat diet, which is the standard recommendation these days, such high-fat foods as olives, olive oil, avocadoes, raw nuts and seeds are frowned upon. But looking at the research and understanding how foods affect your body hormonally, you may look at dietary fat differently now. Let me stress—do not concern yourself too much with healthy dietary fats like monounsaturated and polyunsaturated fats, as they are essential for healthy eicosonoid levels.

Not only are healthy fats important for good eicosonoid production, they also stimulate the release of another important hormone called cholecystokinin or CCK. This hormone affects your appetite control mechanism by signaling meal satiety to the brain. In other words, the release of this hormone makes you feel full. In actuality, this hormone helps prevent the overeating of foods even when considering the extra fat in your diet.

Research shows that moderate-fat, low-processed carbohydrate, adequate-protein meals satisfy hunger much quicker and control appetite much longer than low-fat, high-carbohydrate meals. So, calorie for calorie you not only assist good eicosonoid production with healthy fats and lower processed carbohydrates, but you also promote improved meal satisfaction contributing to less overall food intake.

THE MOST IDEAL DIET FOR OPTIMUM INSULIN AND EICOSONOID LEVELS

The most important method for maintaining ideal insulin and eicosonoid levels is by the foods you eat. Based on the research, a diet that contains adequate protein, low-saturated fats, and very low-processed carbohydrates works best. In other words, optimum health is promoted by eating lots of fresh vegetables, raw nuts and seeds, lean meats and fresh fruits. The most ideal lean meats are fish and fowl.

IN THE NEXT CHAPTER

Hopefully you are more enlightened about how foods affect the quality of your health, risks of disease and life span. By studying our ancestors'diet and understanding the relationship between food and hormonal balance, you are better equipped to make more empowering food choices. Combine this with an earnest desire to improve your overall well-being and you control the destiny of your health. In the next chapter, I will discuss healthy meal options as well as outline a daily menu. I will also tackle some of the more controversial issues such as fat intake, high protein diets and vegetarianism. So, stayed tuned for more on what to eat.

Chapter 6

FOOD FOR THOUGHT

"Are you digging your own grave with a fork?"
ANONYMOUS

One key to a healthy diet is balancing the intake of the three macronutrients: protein, fat and carbohydrates. I will present eating programs in two different formats. First, I will take a more scientific approach for those who are particular about measuring their protein, carbohydrate and fat intake. On the other hand, for those who do not like the complexities of counting calories, carbohydrates, fat, and protein, I will use a more simplistic approach where I suggest foods, meals and eating patterns.

HOW MUCH PROTEIN?

How much protein should I eat? Well, the amount of protein you need is very specific and personalized to your individual body weight and activity level. In fact, if you know your body weight and ascertain your activity level, then you can reliably calculate your daily protein requirement. To get your body weight, simply weigh yourself on an accurate scale first thing in the morning without shoes. To determine your activity level, correlate the amount of physical activity you do to the corresponding activity quotient in Figure 6.1.

FIGURE 6.1

Physical Activity Level	Activity Quotient (Factor to Multiply by Your Body Weight)
Sedentary	.30
Light fitness such as walking 1 to 2 days a week	.40
Moderate physical activity 3 to 4 days a week	.50
Daily aerobic or weight training	.60
Heavy daily weight training or vigorous aerobic activity	.70
Weight training or aerobic exercise twice a day	.80

To help you figure out your activity quotient, let me give you some examples. If you are sedentary or inactive, then your activity quotient is 0.3. If you exercise less than 30 minutes, 1 to 2 times a week, then your activity quotient is 0.4. If you are moderately active or exercise for more than 30 minutes, 3 to 4 times a week, then your activity quotient is 0.5. If you are very physically active or exercise for more than an hour, 5 or 6 days a week, then your activity quotient is 0.6. If you are extremely physically active or are involved in heavy exercise or athletic conditioning more than an hour and a half, 5 or more days a week, then 0.7 is your activity quotient.

Once you figure your individual activity quotient, simply multiply that number times your body weight. The resulting number is your daily protein requirement. It's that simple. Now, to figure how much protein you need for each meal, just divide your daily protein requirement by how many times a day you eat. If, for example, you need 100 grams of protein a day and eat 3 main meals and a snack, then divide 100 by 4. In this case, you should strive to get around 25 grams of protein for each meal and snack. You may choose, however, to get more protein during your main meals and less during your lighter snack. That's okay, just as long as you consume enough protein to meet your daily requirement.

Let me give you some specific examples of calculating protein requirements. Sally, who is a mother and housewife, is active with household chores like cleaning, gardening and tending the kids but doesn't exercise regularly. Her activity quotient would therefore be 0.4 (see Figure 6.1). To calculate her protein needs, simply multiply 0.4 times her body weight, which is 130 pounds. The resulting number is 52, meaning Sally's daily protein requirement is 52 grams. If she eats 4 times a day, then her protein requirement is around 13 grams for each meal or snack.

In another example, John works 5 days a week for a local delivery company, lifting and toting parcels all day long. He doesn't exercise, nor does he actively engage in any physically demanding hobbies. Therefore, his activity quotient is 0.5. Since John weighs 190 pounds, his daily protein intake should be approximately 95 grams (0.5 times 190 = 95). If John eats 5 times a day, he needs around 19 grams of protein for each meal.

And lastly, Janet is training for an upcoming triathlon. She jogs 30 to 50 minutes, 5 to 6 days a week, and lifts weights for nearly 45 minutes twice a week. Therefore, her activity quotient is 0.7. Janet weighs 118 pounds and eats approximately 6 times a day. Accordingly, Janet needs almost 14 grams of protein for each meal. Calculating your personalize protein requirement is that simple and is definitely worth the effort. In fact, knowing your protein requirement is as important as knowing your cholesterol level or blood pressure. You do know what your cholesterol is, don't you?

HOW MUCH FAT?

Now let's go over that three-letter word—FAT. Our society does a remarkable job of being intimidated about the dangers of eating fat. Fat is bad, most people say. Eating it is the reason you get fat, and it is blamed for our society's poor health—or so many believe. Well, I say, "&#@&!>#@&"! After spending 25 years as a conditioning coach and personal trainer and reading literally hundreds of nutrition books, I have found the subject of fat to be one of the most misunderstood topics in the health field.

Nutritionally speaking, if you were to eliminate fat totally from your diet, like most dieters attempt to do, you would die. That's right—die! You need a certain amount of fat to live. In fact, fat is essential. The real problem with our nation's eating habits is not the fat intake per se but the excessive amount of processed foods consumed along with our total calorie intake.

So my advice to you is—DON'T COUNT FAT GRAMS! As a matter of fact, you are going to need some healthy fat in your diet for optimum health. And get this—dietary fat is required in order for you to lose body fat. What—eat fat to lose fat? Are you crazy? (I probably am, but that's beside the point.) The key to burning body fat on a cellular level is to access fat from your adipose tissue. And the access of this fat is promoted by series 1 eicosonoids (the good guys), which is directly dependent on the amount of healthy fat within your diet. Sure, exercise and other factors affect the fat-burning process, but on a cellular level it's the good eicosonoids that stimulate the reduction of your fat cells.

So again, it takes healthy dietary fat to burn body fat. That doesn't mean you can eat all the fat in the world, but it does mean you will have more freedom to consume tastier and more satisfying foods. Don't forget—fat is not the nutritional enemy. As a matter of fact, fat is really the most important component in the flavor of foods. I know sugar tastes good, but fat adds flavor to foods. It also provides longer-lasting satiety and doesn't stimulate your appetite like sugars do. Just think—salads with rich creamy dressings, raw nuts, cheese omelets and foods cooked in olive oil.

Here are some dietary fat recommendations that will help you have healthier eating. When eating meat, simply trim off the visible fat. I recommend using olive oil for all or at least most of your cooking needs and especially for salad dressings. Speaking of olive oil, the Mediterranean diet relies heavily on olive oil, and medical science feels that is one of the reasons their culture has a lower incidence of heart disease and circulatory problems. If you want nuts and seeds, which I recommend, make sure they are raw. The heating or roasting process for most nuts and seeds changes the makeup of the oil to a more harmful compound that can elevate bad eicosonoid production.

The healthiest nuts in terms of monounsaturated fat content and good eicosonoid production are macadamia nuts, walnuts and almonds. The avocado and the olive, which are technically fruits, also contain a high percentage of healthy monounsaturated fat that is very advantageous to your health. The body needs these kinds of fats, especially for their linoleic acid contribution, which, if you recall, is essential for good eicosonoid production.

To sum up, you need 30 percent of your total caloric intake in the form of fat—healthy fat, that is. If you are into counting fat grams, between 30 to 60 grams of healthy fat is a good range. This may seem like an extremely high-fat diet, but I assure you, if you lower your processed carbohydrates and consume healthy fats, you will lose weight and your blood chemistry (cholesterol, HDLs, LDLs, and triglycerides) will definitely improve! What are healthy fats? Healthy fats are unsaturated oils found in nuts, seeds, olives, avocados, and especially fish. The kinds of fats to be minimized or avoided altogether are the saturated kind such as animal fats (four-legged animals have the least desirable fats), dairy fats and especially deep-fried foods or heat-altered fats.

HOW MANY CARBOHYDRATES SHOULD I EAT?

Okay, now let's talk about carbohydrate intake. After much of the information in this chapter points to a low-carbohydrate intake—specifically processed carbohydrates—you might be a little apprehensive about eating carbohydrates or feel they are now the bad guys. Well, they are not the nutritional enemy either, and you don't need to go to the extreme of "zero carbs." Your carbohydrate intake should be between 75 to 125 grams a day. Please keep in mind that almost all of your carbohydrate intake should come from vegetables and fresh fruits. (Didn't your mom tell you to eat that stuff when you were a kid?) If you're not into measuring your food, simply eat vegetables, preferably salads, with every meal except breakfast. Breakfast and snacks are the ideal times to eat fresh fruit. Carbohydrate eating is that simple.

There are many popular diets that now preach low-carbohydrate intake, with some as low as 20 grams per day. But my in-depth research shows optimum nutritional health is achieved, in part, by eating plenty of green vegetables and fresh fruits every day. My research also shows that minimizing the consumption of refined grains and cutting out processed carbohydrates is just as important as eating the right carbohydrates. Remember, it is the amount of processed carbohydrates that negatively affect your insulin levels and eicosonoid production, which ultimately affects your health.

WHAT IS A PROCESSED CARBOHYDRATE?

Throughout Section II, we saw the term processed carbohydrates and how they should be minimized for optimum health. Let me define what

I mean by processed carbohydrates. Processed carbohydrates are products that contain white flour and/or refined sugar as a primary ingredient. This includes most breads, pasta, candy, chips and sugary drinks. A more scientific definition is carbohydrate-rich foods that have been chemically or mechanically changed. For example, french fries are processed potatoes. Cornflakes or corn chips are processed corn. Bread, bagels and pasta are processed wheat. Soda pop is just sugar water with flavor. French fries, chips, white bread, bagels, plain pasta and soft drinks are all primary examples of processed carbohydrates. The success of your eating program will greatly depend on your ability to eliminate or reduce these foods from your diet.

Therefore, I recommend that you limit your intake of processed carbohydrates to less than 30 grams a day. That's the approximate equivalent to a can of soda pop or a standard candy bar or a double-scoop ice cream cone. If you want to lose extra fat or are dissatisfied with your current health, then your processed carbohydrate intake should be less than 10 grams a day. Better yet, cut all processed carbs. A simple trick that will slow the absorption of processed carbohydrates into your bloodstream is to eat them at the end of a healthy meal or snack. This will help minimize the insulin surge and thus lessen the production of bad eicosonoids.

PRACTICAL CARBOHYDRATE EATING

The goal of your eating program is to get the most bang for your buck when choosing your carbohydrates. Vegetables and fruits are the most efficient carbohydrates you can eat because of their fiber content and the ample amount of vitamins, minerals, natural enzymes and powerful phytonutrient qualities they contain. I recommend you consume at least 30 grams of fiber per day, which can be easily accomplished by eating vegetables or fruits at every meal and snack. Even by cutting out a majority of grains from your diet, you will get enough fiber by consuming the recommended vegetables and fruits along with nuts and seeds. Not all carbohydrates are a hindrance to our health, just the inefficient ones, which, ironically, are the most processed.

If you do not want to mess around with counting carbohydrates, I recommend that you eat fresh fruit with breakfast and eat a green salad or other fibrous vegetable with every other meal. Furthermore, minimize or eliminate processed carbohydrates such as breads, pasta, candy, desserts, soda pop and chips from your diet. Or at least substitute lesser-processed carbohydrates for the more processed ones. For example, choose whole wheat bread instead of white bread or whole brown rice over white rice. Even if you can't eliminate processed carbohydrates altogether, at least avoid them on a regular basis. If you reduce dietary processed carbohydrates while maintaining proper fat and protein intake, I promise you will notice a remarkable difference in how you look and feel. You will especially notice a difference in how much looser your clothes will fit and how improved your mood will be. I guarantee it!

ALCOHOLIC BEVERAGES

What about alcohol? Even though alcohol is chemically a carbohydrate, it is digested much differently than other carbohydrates. Alcohol, particularly liquor and beer, raises blood sugar levels, thus increasing insulin response and decreasing good eicosonoid production. All of this has a very negative effect on your overall health. Wine, on the other hand, does have some therapeutic qualities, even though it increases insulin levels. Some wines, particularly red wine, decrease the production of bad eicosonoids, which contributes to increased blood levels of HDLs (the good cholesterol) and lower levels of LDLs (bad cholesterol). Light to moderate consumption of red wine is also linked to decreasing the risks of heart disease and heart attack. The bottom line is one to two glasses of red wine a day may be beneficial to your health. My advice is, if you drink alcoholic beverages, choose red wine and drink it in moderation. I also suggest that you minimize or avoid altogether beer and hard liquor consumption.

THE CARBO-HOLIC

Some of you may be thinking how difficult it is eliminating processed carbohydrates from your diet is going to be. And there are some of you who just do not want to give them up for anything. Let's take bread, for instance. If bread is low in fat and ranks high on the recommended food pyramid, why should I reduce my intake? After all, it is one of society's established healthy foods, right? Well, not according to your body's hormonal response. You may want to reconsider how much of this starch you are eating on a regular basis. Again let me stress, it is not the fat content as much as it is the processed carbohydrates that affect your eicosonoid and insulin levels. If cutting down on processed carbohydrates like breads and pasta seems too difficult, then I suggest following the principles in Chapter 11 on THOUGHT, which outlines how to effectively change habits by self-programming your subconscious mind. But please finish this chapter first.

I used to feel the same way about breads and especially sweets before I fully understood the effect of food on our hormonal balance and ultimately our health. In fact, I used to love sweets, desserts and sugary junk food probably more than a sweet-tooth addict. I loved to eat sugary foods when I was happy, but I craved them more when I was feeling down. Either way, eating sugary junk food made me feel good, at least for a while. A good example of my love for sugary foods was when I used to coach on the collegiate level. When our football team would lose, I would be so dejected and depressed that I would sometimes drown my sorrows, not by drinking alcohol but by consuming a whole ice cream cake roll in one sitting. Now if you know what an ice cream cake roll is, you know that eating one is a real feat. This became almost like an addiction for me. If I wanted to feel better, all I needed to do was eat sweets—and a lot of them!

But I soon began to realize my dairy-delight binges were fast becoming an emotional crutch. You see, I think processed carbohydrates, particularly sweets, are a lot like alcohol or drugs to some people. They can be addictive. I know because I was hooked. I was what you might call a "carbo-holic"—one who is addicted to processed carbohydrates. A lot of people don't realize it, but they are carbo-holics, too. But how do you know? Can you give up breads and sweets for a week? A month? If not, you may be a carbo-holic. To achieve optimum health and be totally fit, the carbohydrate addiction must be stopped.

One of the best ways to break this carbohydrate addiction was demonstrated over 30 years ago by three medical doctors and is still used today, especially in the bodybuilding field. Dr's Pennington, Atkins, and Bloom successfully showed on different occasions that eating only proteins and fats with very little carbohydrates (less than 20 grams a day) for a week forces the body to burn fat as energy instead of glucose. Glucose, if you recall, is a simple sugar derived from carbohydrates and is the preferred fuel of your brain. However, in the absence of dietary carbohydrates, the body is eventually forced to generate substitute energy molecules called ketone bodies from the available fats stores. Using ketone bodies as an energy source is very inefficient and may present some health concerns. I recommend this sort of carbohydrate-restricted diet for only severely overweight individuals. Nevertheless, it is one alternative for eliminating the sugar addiction.

However, I recommend a safer, more practical method for tossing the sugar-monkey off your back. And it rids body fat to boot. This "carbo-busting" strategy eliminates all processed carbohydrates for three days. It is not, however, a zero-carbohydrate plan. That's the difference—a healthy difference. Even though I suggest eliminating all fruits and juices (only for three days) to cut carbs, it is imperative that you eat green fibrous vegetables during this sugar-busting period. This three-day, carbo-buster meal plan consist of eating only lean meats, nuts, seeds and raw green salads. And I do mean plenty of salads.

Many of my clients, including myself, have participated in this three-day eating scheme and found the results amazing. Eliminating all processed carbohydrates and fruits for 72 hours isn't as difficult as you think, and the rewards are absolutely tremendous. For me, it has been more than two years since that carbohydrate-kicking three days, and I haven't had any of those nasty sugar cravings or junk food binges since. And isn't that the key? Once you reduce your processed carbohydrate intake, you will notice a drastic reduction in your cravings for unhealthy sweets and processed foods. But the biggest advantages, besides fat loss, are the long-term benefits of being a healthier individual.

SALADS AND FRESH FRUITS ARE THE KEY

As far as vegetables are concerned, eat as much as you want. *Fresh green salads are the key to this dietary program and are probably the very best food(s) you can eat.* My favorite salads often contain nuts or seeds or even lean chicken or turkey breast. One of the reasons green salads are so healthy and beneficial is the fact they are eaten raw. And eating raw vegetables and fruits allows the body to get more of the natural enzymes, vitamins, minerals and special phytonutrients that are usually destroyed by cooking or processing. Although cooked vegetables are okay, the living phytochemical and natural enzymes in these raw foods aid human digestion and promote better health. As added kudos, salads will now taste better, because you can use any salad dressing you like, especially those containing olive oil. As I said earlier, don't worry about the unsaturated fats found in salad dressings.

A note on fruits. Most nutritionists will tell you to eat all the fruit you can. But quite frankly, eating too much fruit can affect the sugar storage in your liver, which ultimately affects your body fat levels. Also, too much fruit may trigger carbohydrate cravings, since they contain mostly sugar, even though it's a healthy sugar. One to two servings of fresh fruit a day is okay. The best fruits are apples, pears, cantaloupe, melons and berries because they have lower sugar and higher fiber compared to other fruits. Apples and pears are especially beneficial since they contain valuable pectin as their main fiber.

THE RECOMMENDED EATING PLAN

So, to sum up, I recommend the following: Eat low-saturated-fat proteins at every meal such as fish, fowl, eggs, other lean meats, low-fat cottage cheese, plain yogurt, raw nuts and seeds. (If you eat yogurt, I recommend natural, unsweetened, plain yogurt. This type of yogurt has more beneficial bacteria and enzymes and less sugar. Most fruit-flavored yogurts have over 50 grams of carbohydrates per serving, which is too much.) Eat a green salad or other green vegetables with every meal, except breakfast, such as a tossed green salad, broccoli, asparagus, sprouts, celery and so on. Eat fresh, raw fruit before your breakfast meal and as a snack. Try to eat fruit on an empty stomach for better digestion.

If you are a calorie counter, my research shows that the most beneficial and life-enhancing diet should provide between 1,200 to 1,800 calories per day. Of all the controversy surrounding the nutrition field, there is one premise that's unanimously accepted: eating less than 1,500 calories a day maximizes your health and extends your life dramatically. But the real key to a low-calorie diet is the macronutrient makeup. I recommend 30 percent protein, 40 percent carbohydrates (low processed) and 30 percent fat (healthy fat, that is). After you pull yourself off the floor from seeing the fat intake, let me remind you it's the healthy fat and not the bad kind (saturated) that I recommend. There is a difference! But don't take my word for it. Check your body fat and blood chemistry after six weeks of eating this way and see for yourself. It really does work!

FIGURE 6.2 SAMPLE MENU

Breakfast	Apple, pear, orange, grapefruit, berries or any other fresh fruit *and* Cheese omelet or egg whites and/or Canadian bacon or plain yogurt or cottage cheese
Lunch	Chicken Caesar salad (without croutons), Cobb salad, tossed salad, Chinese chicken salad, tuna salad, or create your own green salad with lean meat
Snack	Low-fat cottage cheese with fruit, or macadamia nuts, or fresh fruit, or raw walnuts, or fruit and cheese, or raw vegetables, or plain yogurt, or peanut butter and celery sticks
Dinner	Grilled chicken, baked pork chops, lean steak, stir-fry chicken, baked salmon, cooked cod, or sliced turkey breast *and* Large green dinner salad, steamed broccoli with cheese, cooked asparagus, or stir-fry vegetables

Dinner, lunch and even breakfast foods can be interchangeable. For example, you could have a vegetable omelet for dinner or fresh fruit and salmon for breakfast. Be creative, and have fun putting together a healthy menu. Just remember that the key is to eat low-saturated-fat proteins with each meal, along with fresh raw fruit at breakfast and a green salad or vegetable at lunch and dinner. Raw nuts and seeds, plain yogurt or fruit and cheese serve as ideal snacks.

Figure 6.3 shows one day's menu on a low-calorie program (less than 1,500 calories). You can see that it is healthy, filling and at the same time adequate in healthy fats.

Notice how the macronutrients are divided in terms of percentage of calories (30 percent protein, 40 percent carbohydrates and 30 percent fat). However, according to most of today's accepted dietary guidelines, the fat intake and percentage of fat to total calories in this particular menu would be too high. But if you truly understand your body's hormonal response to food and how the proper balance of macronutrients produces good eicosonoid levels, then you can appreciate this higher healthy fat and lower carbohydrate menu. Please note how low the daily total calories are, even though many would call this a high-fat diet. But remember, a low-calorie (less than 1,500) menu containing adequate protein, low processed carbohydrates and plenty of healthy fats is a must for good eicosonoid production and overall health. Furthermore, even though no processed breads or grains are consumed, the fiber intake is 43 grams, which exceeds the daily (RDA) recommendation of 25 grams. But the most important category shows only 6 grams of processed carbohydrates being consumed. This is well below the daily 30-gram intake limit that I recommend for processed carbohydrates.

FIGURE 6.3 TYPICAL DAILY MENU

	Calories	Proteins	Carbs	Fats	Fiber	Processed Carbohydrates
BREAKFAST Strawberries 1 1/2 cups Cheese/mushroom omelet w/olive oil & Egg Beaters Whole wheat toast with jam						
Meal Total	**400**	**29**	**39**	**14**	**11**	**0**
LUNCH Mixed green salad w/turkey breast, bleu cheese dressing, celery, tomato, cucumber, romaine, onion with whole wheat croutons						
Meal Total	**422**	**32**	**44**	**13**	**12**	**0**
SNACK Flavored Soy Nuts 1 medium apple						
Meal Total	**201**	**12**	**30**	**4**	**8**	**0**
DINNER Baked Salmon, 5 oz w/ Hollandaise sauce Grilled asparagus Green salad Whole wheat bread Glass of Merlot wine						
Meal Total	**475**	**38**	**49**	**14**	**12**	**6**
Grand Total	Calories	Proteins	Carbs	Fats	Fiber	Processed Carbohydrates
Daily Total	**1,498**	**111**	**162**	**45**	**43**	**6 (from the wine)**
% of Diet		**30%**	**43%**	**27%**		

VITAMINS AND MINERALS

Even though consuming fresh green salads, raw nuts and seeds, healthy proteins and in-season fruits is the best way of achieving optimum nutrition, I encourage you to take a quality multiple vitamin and mineral supplement regularly. Until just recently, most nutritionists believed that a proper diet delivered all the essential nutrients without having to rely on supplementation. However, current medical data shows that most people do not get all the nutrients they need from the foods they eat. For example, an extensive 14-year study following 80,000 women found that nearly 90 percent were deficient in several essential vitamins, namely B6, B12 and folic acid. In another study, 40 percent of patients who had hip fractures were deficient in vitamin D. Furthermore, research shows that nutritional deficiencies are most prevalent among the elderly.

But the real key to vitamin and mineral intake, especially in people over 40, is absorption. It is estimated that only 10 to 12 percent of the adults who take vitamin and mineral supplements fully absorb them. Processed carbohydrates, caffeine, alcohol, certain medications, smoking, stress and aging all affect the absorption of these vital nutrients. Furthermore, as people grow older, extraction of essential nutrients during digestion becomes less efficient due to reduced stomach acidity and a less absorbent intestinal lining.

However, I do not suggest taking higher dosages of vitamins and minerals as a method of overcoming insufficient nutrient absorption. As a matter of fact, taking too much of certain vitamins and minerals can be harmful to your health. But what's the best way of getting the proper amount of necessary nutrients effectively into your bloodstream? The answer is liquid or dissolvable powder vitamins and minerals. Of all the vitamin and mineral supplements that I have evaluated for my clients and athletes, I personally recommend taking vitamins and minerals in a liquid or dissolvable powder form. It is the optimum way for vitamins and minerals to be absorbed.

Medical reports and the Physician's Desk Reference state that 90 to 95 percent of the nutrients in liquid or dissolvable powder form are absorbed within 30 seconds after consuming. Tablets, capsules, and gel caps, on the other hand, are less than 30 percent absorbed. (Most are 5 to 20 percent absorbed.) In the future, more and more drugs and medications will be administered by this new, very effective delivery system. The bottom line is, make sure you eat right to achieve maximum nutrient absorption and "drink" your vitamins and minerals everyday.

WHAT ABOUT VEGETARIANS?

Another question on eating that provokes conflicting opinions is the consumption of meat and animal products. Let me address the issue of vegetarianism because some of you may be vegetarians or know people who are. I can speak from personal experience on this topic, since I was a strict vegan for almost two years. A vegan consumes grains, vegetables, fruits, nuts and seeds but no animal products such as meat, dairy and eggs. Lacto-ovo vegetarians may eat eggs and dairy products in addition to grains, vegetables, fruits, nuts and seeds.

Following a strict vegan program and consuming no animal products, I physically felt pretty good and experienced no noticeable health problems during those two years. Of course, I was exercising daily and following many of the health principles I would later write about in this book. However, during my first year of coaching with the U.S. Ski team, I had the opportunity to participate in a protein study that was being done on some of our Olympic athletes. This study involved nitrogen balance measurements to determine if our athletes were consuming enough protein for their activity level. Even though I was not an aspiring Olympic athlete, I was into health and wanted to prove, especially to my athletes, how abstaining from animal products was truly beneficial and healthy. Since I was the only vegetarian participant in this study and truly believed in my way of eating, I couldn't wait to disprove the theory that so many coaches and athletes held on eating large amounts of protein.

The nitrogen balance test works by measuring the amount of nitrogen you excrete through your urine and feces and comparing it to the amount of nitrogen you consume. Since dietary protein is the only source of nitrogen, simply calculating the amount of protein you eat versus the amount of nitrogen you excrete shows how much protein your body is utilizing. If you excrete more measurable nitrogen than you take in through your diet, then you are in a negative nitrogen balance, meaning you are not consuming enough dietary protein. If, on the other hand, you consume more protein than you excrete, you are in a positive nitrogen balance, meaning you are eating more protein than your body needs. From a true health standpoint, nitrogen balance should measure near zero or slightly above, meaning you are consuming enough protein to satisfy your body's needs.

As far as human health is concerned, a prolonged negative nitrogen balance can prove unhealthy and even harmful. It has been observed in almost every disease state, a negative nitrogen balance exists indicating how important adequate protein absorption is to one's overall health. In fact, extensive studies on nitrogen balance and physical activity contributed to the scientific data found in Figure 6.1 that you utilized while calculating your individual protein requirement.

Now that I have explained the premise behind the nitrogen balance test, let's get back to the protein study performed on the Olympic athletes and myself. To my complete surprise, the test results showed that I was in a negative nitrogen balance, meaning I was not eating enough dietary protein to sustain my physical activity level. Thinking all along that abstaining from meat and animal protein contributed to optimum health proved to be wrong in my case. That, my friend, is the reason I no longer subscribe to being a vegetarian. I'm not against following vegetarianism, but I encourage you to be aware of consuming enough protein for your body's activity level if you are a vegetarian. So, make sure you use the information in Figure 6.1 to determine your individual protein needs.

MY PERSONAL STORY

Nutrition is like politics and religion in that most people have a definite opinion about the subject, and many feel they are "experts." Well, I tried to be unbiased and forego my educational background while restudying this very controversial health topic. I made every attempt to approach the nutrition field like an open-minded detective searching for evidence and clues on how humans are designed to eat. Without a doubt, the eating recommendations in this book may be controversial, but they do indeed work, not just for fat loss but for overall improved cellular health.

Before I started the extensive nutritional research for this chapter, I scoffed at the lower-carbohydrate, higher-unsaturated-fat concept. It just didn't jive with the conventional wisdom of today's nutritional philosophy. But now that I have analyzed the compelling arguments and overwhelming evidence, there is no doubt this is the dietary program for me. In fact, after four months of following this eating plan, my body fat percentage dropped from 19 percent to less than 10 percent, and my waist-line decreased 3 1/2 inches.

The best thing about eating this way is that my mood and energy level have been phenomenal. Writing a book containing nutritional recommendations that are so against what I was taught in college and have firmly believed for years shows how much I believe in these eating principles. I may not have a PhD in nutrition, but I have a PhD in results.

SUMMARY

I must admit that before starting the research for this chapter, I was not sold on a moderate-protein, low-processed-carbohydrate, healthy-fat diet. My initial lack of conviction is indeed what allowed me to perform a more diligent quest to find the answers to some of the most basic nutrition questions. Mainly, how are humans supposed to eat? With all my coaching, personal training, and even individual experience relating to this very controversial subject, there is no doubt in my mind that this plan will deliver the most optimum health benefits possible. Simply follow these dietary principles, and I am sure you will marvel at the positive transformation that your physical body will experience and that your overall health will undergo. Good luck and good eating!

HEALTH HABIT 9:

Eat adequate low-fat protein sources such as fish, chicken, turkey, eggs, cottage cheese, beef and plain yogurt daily. The amount of dietary protein intake should be specific and individualized for your lean body weight and activity level. See Figure 6.1 to calculate your lean weight and activity level.

HEALTH HABIT 8:

Consume a fresh green salad or fibrous vegetable with every meal except breakfast. Fresh green garden salads are probably the healthiest food you can consume. Fibrous vegetables include asparagus, broccoli, lettuce, carrots, celery, cucumber, spinach, artichoke, cabbage, cauliflower, kale, mushrooms, sprouts, peppers and tomatoes. Also consume onions and garlic regularly.

HEALTH HABIT 7:

Consume fresh fruit with breakfast and as a snack. Eat fresh fruits in their whole, natural state. Recommended fresh fruits are apples, apricots, berries, cantaloupe, cherries, grapefruit, grapes, melon, kiwi, nectarines, oranges, peaches, pears, pineapple, plums, tangerines and watermelon.

HEALTH HABIT 6:

Minimize or avoid processed carbohydrate consumption such as white breads, plain pasta, sweets, pastries, muffins, candy, sugary drinks, soda pop, chips, processed cereals and cookies.

REFERENCE OUT TAKES

On Cancer

"Saturated fat was not associated with the risk of breast cancer. We found no positive association between intake of total fat and risk of invasive breast cancer."

—A. Wolk, et al., *Archives of Internal Medicine*, 1998, 158: 41-45.

"We found no evidence of a positive association between total dietary fat intake and the risk of breast cancer. There was no reduction in risk even among women whose energy intake from fat was less than 20 percent of total energy intake. In the context of the Western lifestyle, lowering the total intake of fat in mid-life is unlikely to reduce the risk of breast cancer substantially."

—D. Hunter, et al., *New England Journal of Medicine*, 1996.

"Sugar consumption is positively associated with cancer in humans and test animals. Tumors are known to be enormous sugar absorbers."

—Sally Fallon, *Nourishing Traditions*, 1995 Promotion Publishing. Joseph D. Beasley, MD and Jerry J. Swift, MA, *The Kellogg Report*, 1989, The Institute of Healthy Policy and Practice, Annandale-on-Hudson, New York, 129.

"Johns Hopkins researchers have found evidence that some cancer cells are such incredible sugar junkies that they'll self-destruct when deprived of glucose, their biological sweet of choice. Scientists have long suspected that the cancer cell's heavy reliance on glucose, its main source of strength and vitality, also could be one of its great weaknesses, and Dang's new results are among the most direct proofs yet of the idea."

—Johns Hopkins Medical Institutions' news release. H. Shim and C. Dang, *Proceedings of the National Academy of Sciences* USA, Feb. 17, 1998, 95(4): 1511-1516.

On Cardiovascular Disease

"Abnormalities in glucose and insulin metabolism are commonly found in patients with high blood pressure. There is evidence suggesting that defects in glucose and insulin metabolism may play a role in both the origin and the natural history of high blood pressure."

—G. Reaven, et al., *The American Journal of Medicine*, 1989, 87(supp 6A): 6A-2S.

"More plagues than heart disease can be laid at sugar's door. A survey of medical journals in the 1970s produced findings implicating sugar as a causative factor in kidney disease, liver disease, shortened life span, increased desire for coffee and tobacco, as well as arteriosclerosis and coronary heart disease."

—Sally Fallon, *Nourishing Traditions*, 1995 Promotion Publishing. Edward Howell, MD, *Enzyme Nutrition*, 1985, Avery Publishing, Inc.

On Diabetes

"These results suggest that a high-protein, low-carbohydrate diet, with nutritional supplementation can be useful to reduce several cardiovascular risk factors in obese adult onset diabetic patients including weight, blood sugar and lipid parameters. There is also no evidence that the nutritional regimen adversely affects kidney function."

—J.S. Edman, et al., *Journal of the American College of Nutrition*, October 1998.

"It seems prudent to avoid the use of low-fat, high-carbohydrate diets containing moderate amounts of sucrose in patients with non-insulin-dependent diabetes mellitus."

—A. M. Coulston, et al., *American Journal of Medicine*, Feb. 1987, 82(2): 213-220.

"As compared with high-carbohydrate diets, the high-monounsaturated-fat diet resulted in lower mean plasma glucose levels and reduced insulin requirements, lower levels of plasma triglycerides and very low-density lipo-protein cholesterol and higher levels of high-density lipoprotein (good cholesterol). Levels of total cholesterol did not differ significantly in patients on the two diets."

—A. Garg, et al., *New England Journal of Medicine*, 1998, 319 (13): 829-834.

On Stroke

"Intakes of fat, saturated fat, and monosaturated fat were associated with reduced risk of ischemic stroke in men." (From the Framingham Heart Study)

—M. Gillman, et al., *Journal of the American Medical Association*, 1997, 78(24): 2145-2150.

On the Low-Fat Diet

"Low-fat diets low in polyunsaturated fatty acids induce essential fatty acid (EFA) insufficiency, and can increase the biochemical risk factors for heart disease: they may also increase appetite."

—E. Siguel, *BioMedicina*, January 1998, 1(1): 9.

"Low-fat, high-carbohydrate diets also reduce high-density lipoprotein (good cholesterol) levels and raise fasting levels of triglycerides."

—R. P. Mensink, et al., *Arteriorsclet Thomb*, Aug. 1992, 12(8): 911-919.

"The relative good health of the Japanese, who have the longest life span in the world, is generally attributed to a low-fat diet. Those who point to Japanese statistics to promote the low-fat diet fail to mention that the Swiss live almost as long on one of the fattiest diets in the world. Tied for third in longevity are Austria and Greece—both with high-fat diets."

—Sally Fallon, *Nourishing Traditions*, 1995 Promotion Publishing. Thomas J. Moore, *Life Span: What Really Affects Human Longevity*, 1990, Simon & Schuster, New York.

"There is still the potential for low-fat intakes to adversely affect the nutritional adequacy of the diet of children. Given the assumption that there are some potential nutritional dangers associated with the unsupervised use of such diets, with no proven benefits, this diet should definitely not be advocated for infants and young children."

—S. H. Zlotkin, *Arch Pediatr Adolesc Med*, 1997, 151: 962-963.

"In 1821, the average sugar intake in America was 10 pounds per person per year; today it is 170 pounds per person, over one-fourth the average caloric intake. Another large fraction of all calories comes from refined flour and refined vegetable oils."

—Sally Fallon, *Nourishing Traditions*, 1995 Promotion Publishing. Joseph D. Beasley, MD and Jerry J. Swift, MA, *The Kellogg Report*, 1989, The Institute of Health Policy and Practice, Annadale-on-Hudson, New York, 144-145.

"A recent study involving over 40,000 middle-aged and older American men over a six-year period found that there was no link between saturated fat intake and heart disease in men. It also supported the contention that linolenic acid (a form of fat) is preventive against heart disease."

—A. Ascherio, et al., Dietary fat and risk of coronary heart disease in men: cohort follow-up study in the United States. *British Medical Journal*, Jul. 13, 1996, 313:7049, 84-90.

"In a two-year study, 171 women on a low-fat diet achieved a maximum weight loss of only about seven and a half pounds at 6 months, and by year two some of that weight was regained. Most significantly, the standard deviation was more than twice the average weight loss, showing that a number of subjects actually gained weight on the low-fat diet, not counting the 13 that dropped out of the program."

—L. Sheppard, et al., Weight Loss in Women Participating in a Randomized Trial of Low-Fat Diets. *American Journal of Clinical Nutrition*, 1991, 54: 821-828.

SECTION III

SLEEP

"Anything that can't be done in bed isn't something worth doing at all."

GROUCHO MARX

Chapter 7

WAKE ME WHEN I'M WELL

"Sleep's the only medicine that gives ease."
SOPHOCLES

In the mid-1980s, while I was coaching at the University of Utah, I remember talking to the Air Force strength coach at midfield prior to the kickoff of the Air Force-Utah football game. On this particular occasion, we were talking about the latest training principles many college and professional sports programs use to improve athletic performance. I am always eager to hear other ideas and philosophies from the various strength coaches around the country about the best ways to achieve optimal physical conditioning. Oh, the usual diet and weight training programs are typically discussed, but something the Air Force strength coach revealed that beautiful fall day will always stick in my mind.

He explained an interesting concept the Air Force Academy was experimenting with to successfully get their athletes into peak physical condition, and it didn't involve any special weight training program or nutritional supplement. No, it involved a concept much simpler than that. It involved the addition of sleep. Quality, restful sleep, that is. It appeared that, by adding extra sleep to an athlete's daily training program at the appropriate time, remarkable improvements were being observed. Such an elementary concept of improving an athlete's performance by the simple addition of quality sleep was almost too easy to accept. But it actually made sense, nevertheless.

Athletic conditioning coaches spend countless hours mapping out training schedules, formulating exercise regiments, and even prescribing nutritional plans in an all-out effort to build a better athlete. But one of the most important aspects of an athlete's training program is, in fact, one of the least discussed and seldom implemented. And that is adequate, restful, consistent, uninterrupted sleep. As I studied this subject more in depth, it became increasingly apparent how proper sleep principles can affect the training and performance of hard-driving athletes.

But I also found that these same sleep principles could affect more than just diligent training athletes, as I would later observe while personal-training general public clientele. In today's health-conscious world, many books are written on how diet and exercise impact our general health, but very few health programs encompass the integral aspects of the all-important factor of quality sleep.

HOW WE VALUE SLEEP

As it turns out, of all the health principles discussed in this book, sleep is taken for granted the most and is probably understood the least. Our value on sleep as a society is somewhat hypocritical. Most everyone agrees they need adequate, quality sleep, but few place the priority for ample sleep very high on their list of health goals. For the truly busy person, sleep just seems to get in the way. In fact, most top business executives rank getting eight or more hours of sleep as a luxury. "It is one of those necessary things you have to do," a top company CEO recently stated at one of my health workshops.

When I start discussing the subject of sleep in my health seminars, I often hear many participants brag about how little sleep they manage to get, like it's kind of a macho feat. But is getting less sleep really a"cool thing"? In all the latest research on this subject the opposite really should be the case. By understanding the principles of sleep and how it greatly affects your performance in life, you would then be one of those rare healthy individuals bragging about how much quality sleep you were getting.

But the little premium we place on adequate sleep seems justified as one of the ways for coping with the rat race our society has become. Just the other day, I noticed a TV commercial about a large mail delivery company now offering Sunday delivery service. This is just one of the many signs that our society has become a seven-days-a-week, 24-hours-a-day, on-the-go society. And with time at a premium, quality, adequate, restful sleep is usually the activity most sacrificed.

When I worked with the Olympic Ski team, I had the privilege of spending quite a bit of time traveling throughout the alpine countries of Europe. One of the many differences I noticed in most of these far-away regions was the slower pace of life. Some of the amenities our country has come to expect were seldom found during my travels there. For example, there were very few gas stations open late at night, almost no 24-hour convenience stores for midnight sugar-craving Twinkie runs, and the television stations concluded their programming usually before midnight.

Another unfamiliar custom I had only heard about was the closing of most markets and stores for almost two hours every weekday afternoon for what is commonly known as afternoon *siestas*. During my first few stays in Europe, these inconveniences were very frustrating. But I soon learned to accept this slower way of life with more understanding. As of this writing, many European countries are slowly transforming into a busier, more hectic society like ours.

But striving to become a busier society is not without its disadvantages. The price of this jet-paced way of living has most Americans working more hours, participating in more outside activities, and even watching more television, all at the expense of sleep. But I ask you, what is this increasing pinch on the amount of sleep doing to our society's health and quality of life? Do you know what the quality of your life is as the result of less sleep? If you don't, you will after you read this chapter. So, wake up and read, unless it is past your bedtime; otherwise, wait until tomorrow when you are better rested.

ARE YOU GETTING ENOUGH?

How many hours a night should you sleep? Are you getting enough sleep? How do you know if you are getting enough sleep? I have listed 14 statements that will help you determine if you are getting enough sleep. Take the following quiz and see how you stack up. Answer Yes or No to the following statements.

1. I need an alarm clock to wake up at the appropriate time.
2. It is a struggle for me to get out of bed in the morning.
3. Weekday mornings I hit the snooze button several times to get more sleep.
4. I feel more tired, irritable and stressed out during the week compared to weekends.
5. I have trouble concentrating and remembering.
6. I feel slow at times with critical thinking, problem solving and being creative.
7. I often fall asleep watching TV.
8. I often fall asleep in boring meetings or lectures or in warm rooms.
9. I often fall asleep while relaxing after dinner.
10. I often fall asleep within five minutes after going to bed.
11. I often feel drowsy while driving.

12. I often sleep extra hours on weekends.
13. I often need a nap to get through the day.
14. I have dark circles under my eyes (that's pre-makeup).

If you answered yes to more than 3 of the 14 statements, you are not getting enough sleep. You are sleep deprived! Interesting, huh? If you are sleep deprived, you are not alone. A 1995 Gallup poll estimated 100 million Americans are sleep deprived, with one-third of our population sleeping less than 6 hours a night. Our national sleep habits tell us a lot about the many changes taking place in our society. In the early 1900s Americans slept an average of 10 hours per night, and today that average is 6 1/2 hours. So, we have lost more than 3 hours of sleep this century, even though our bodies have not genetically changed during that time. What are the repercussions of this sleep deprivation?

IMPACT ON OUR SOCIETY

Whether you know it or not, everyone is affected by our country's lack of sleep. Studies show that 31 percent of all automobile drivers have fallen asleep while driving during their lifetime. Next time you take a trip, there is a good chance the driver passing you, behind you or even in front of you is sleep deprived. The National Sleep Foundation estimates that 100,000 traffic accidents and 1,500 fatalities occur each year as a result of drivers falling asleep at the wheel. The National Transportation Board says fatigue is the number one detrimental impact on an airline pilot's ability to fly. To relate to this, I read a shockingly true story about an airline pilot who dozed off while copiloting a 747 on a long flight and woke up only to find everyone else in the cockpit asleep. Just think, a 747 with a flying crew all asleep at the helm. That is really frightening, especially if you are reading this book while flying commercially!

What about daylight saving time? How does this seasonal change affect our sleep? Well, a Canadian study gives us a good example on the sobering facts about daylight saving time and how it affects our society. The Monday after the switch to daylight saving time, and one hour of sleep is lost, traffic fatalities increase 7 percent. Oddly enough, the Monday after we go off daylight saving time, where an extra hour of sleep is gained, the statistics show an almost identical change but in reverse. Here highway deaths decrease almost 7 percent. Is daylight saving time really a saving after all when you consider how detrimental just one hour of sleep loss can be on an already sleep-deprived society?

Another problem related to sleep deprivation involves shift workers, especially second and third shift. Most of the workplace problems involving accidents, sickness, and fatigue can be attributed to lack of sleep. The nuclear accidents at Chernoble and Three Mile Island, for example, both occurred in the early morning hours during the third shift. Most of today's work-related accidents and sick days can be indirectly related to sleep deprivation. Over $80 is spent each year by companies dealing with these kinds of work-related problems, estimates the National Sleep Foundation. So, don't tell me you save time by allowing work to cut into your sleep because in the long run you don't save time... or money.

HOW SLEEP LOSS AFFECTS YOU

Working night shifts presents a myriad of concerns for both employers and employees alike, and it affects you, the general public, in more subtle ways than you think. Case in point is the status of our medical care shift workers. Statistically, medical residents, interns and even doctors are the most sleep deprived of all! Just think, the people who are the most responsible for your health and well-being, especially during surgeries and emergencies, are in all likelihood sleep deprived. Some medical care personnel, especially doctors, sometimes work over 130 hours per week, with shifts ranging from 12 to 60 hours. Imagine pulling into the emergency room needing immediate medical attention and the attending physician has been without sleep for 50 hours. A terrifying thought, but it does happen, and it does affect you.

As you can see, it doesn't take a rocket scientist to understand most of us need more sleep, some more than others. Oddly enough, most sleep-deprived individuals have grown so accustomed to being tired and lethargic that they aren't even aware of their need for more sleep. A low energy level or bad mood is usually written off without considering deficient sleep as the possible culprit. For some, however, being aware of their need for sufficient sleep isn't enough to prioritize making it a consistent nightly habit. But if you know you need more sleep, what possible reason or reasons would prevent you from getting it? When I posed that question to many business executives during a recent seminar, the reply was almost unanimous: "I don't have time" or "I am too busy." But sacrificing sleep to accommodate a busy schedule or hectic lifestyle isn't the answer and does prove inefficient in the long run.

The fact is, numerous studies show that inadequate sleep does lead to unproductive work, poor concentration, mental errors, higher susceptibility to accidents and the increase in frequency of illness. The short-term effects of sleep loss may produce nothing more than fatigue, decreased memory, poor emotional disposition and inadequate concentration. But continued sleep deprivation—say, longer than a few days—may expose you to more serious health risks such as accelerated aging, serious accidents and a less efficient immune system.

Yes, even your chances of illness or disease are greatly increased if you experience just minimal sleep loss. That's because your body's immune system is directly related to the amount of sleep you receive. If you lose one hour of sleep on any given night, your immune system decreases 30 percent in effectiveness. This very moment you are exposed to millions of invading bacteria and viruses that your body's immune system is constantly battling. Most of the battles against these foreign intruders are won by your hard-working bug-fighting system. But when you short-change your sleep quota, your immune system has a more difficult time winning these battles, which ultimately contributes to increased sickness and poorer health. In short, the extra time achieving your ideal sleep quota will more than make up for the negative health consequences attributed to inadequate sleep.

WHAT IS SLEEP?

The dictionary defines sleep as "a natural recurring condition of suspended consciousness." Even though science is continuously learning more about this nightly process, sleep still remains very mysterious. Throughout the ages, the enigma about this slumbering state has contributed to old wives' tales and unfounded beliefs. Thomas Edison, the famous inventor and the one who changed our sleep habits the most, was appalled at sleep. He thought it served very little purpose and, for the most part, was a waste of time.

In Edison's biography, it was noted how he would sometimes stay up all night, working on inventions, completely forgetting to sleep. He did believe, nonetheless, that sleep served a useful biological purpose. Since you could not do very much at night with little light, he reasoned this was God's way of telling us to lie down and physically rest the body. Even with the rest, sleep is still something to do just to pass the night away, he would say. In spite of his proclaimed disgust for sleep, he was very notorious for secretly taking naps during the day, especially after staying up all night, working in his laboratory. But sleep is much more than simply passing the night away or resting the physical body, as you will soon see.

Even though this suspended state appears to be a dormant and resting phase, there are a lot of biological activities taking place. When you sleep your overall level of neuron activity drops by only 10 percent. This means the nerve impulses and your ability to transmit messages are almost as active during the sleeping phase as during the waking state. And believe it or not, the brain is actually more active during sleep, even with a 10 percent drop in neuron activity.

The sleeping brain regulates gastrointestinal, cardiovascular and immune functions. The sleeping brain energizes the body. The sleeping brain also organizes and files all new information and develops cognitive processing, which includes reorganization of data already stored. For example, if you study or learn something during the day, that night when you go to sleep your brain is processing that new information. The more quality sleep you get, the more you increase the likelihood of transferring that stored short-term information into long-term memory.

A study involving college students during final exams showed they experienced deeper, longer sleep cycles for several days after taking exams. Their need for extra sleep was attributed to the additional information being processed, absorbed, stored, and transferred into long-term memory by the sleeping brain. Researchers have also found that the proper amount of sleep during the growing years of childhood does contribute to a higher capacity of brain power and cognitive skills later in life. Furthermore, one particular study indicates a child's IQ can be positively affected by the appropriate amount of quality, restful sleep. So, do you still think sleep is a waste of time or just for physical rest?

THE FOUR STAGES OF SLEEP

So what exactly is sleep? Sleep is scientifically divided into four stages or phases. Measurements of brain wave activity, hormonal secretions, neurological impulses and breathing patterns are all involved in helping science classify each of these sleep cycles. One of the first biological events that happen in preparation for sleep can be found in the electromagnetic wavelength changes in the brain. During the waking state, the brain normally produces beta waves, which are longer-frequency electromagnetic waves. But just prior to sleep, as the body becomes more relaxed, the brain's beta wavelengths give way to slower, shorter electrical waves called alpha waves.

These lower-activity alpha waves are associated with a more restful, less tense state. If you recall from Section I, the act of deep, diaphragmatic breathing also produces a calmer, more tranquil emotional state by stimulating these same brain alpha waves. You might say, in a sense, that deep diaphragmatic breathing helps prime the brain by facilitating this electromagnetic wavelength change, thereby dramatically enhancing the initial stages of sleep.

After several minutes of alpha wave electromagnetic activity, the brain waves continue to slow. This happens after a few moments of being in bed before you actually fall asleep. As you start to drift away, your brain wavelengths shorten even more from alpha waves to theta waves. Brain theta waves signify Stage 1 sleep and can last from 10 seconds to 10 minutes. During this initial stage, you feel only half asleep and are still vaguely aware of your environment. Your breathing pattern, heart rate, and other biological functions begin to slow.

During Stage 1 sleep, the cortex of the brain is starting to immobilize the skeletal muscles, so as you slip into deeper sleep you cannot harm yourself with uncontrollable muscular movements. This partial "paralysis" is the reason you do not actually run in bed or move violently, even though you may experience these actions in your dreams. Have you ever been right on the edge of falling asleep and had a sudden muscle jerk or twitch? That's because the brain cortex has not yet completely immobilized the skeletal muscles as they are beginning to relax. This is a normal process and signifies your body is entering the next stage of sleep.

As you descend into Stage 2 sleep, the theta waves now shift into even smaller electromagnetic wavelengths called K waves. You have probably noticed by now that the brain wave activity has been progressively diminishing into lower-frequency wavelengths ever since you closed your eyes. Stage 2 sleep actually marks the beginning of true sleep. At this point you are not cognizant of the activities around you. In fact, you are deaf and blind to all environmental stimuli such as talking, motion and illuminated lights. Muscle tension and nerve impulses are greatly reduced during this sleep phase, which lasts from 10 to 20 minutes.

Okay, it has now been 20 to 30 minutes since you first closed your eyes, having gone through the first two stages of sleep. Now you are about to enter Stage 3 sleep. This third stage of sleep exhibits a gradual shift from theta waves to lower frequency, high-voltage delta waves. During this stage the body and brain continue to slow down in activity. As you proceed into the next sleep phase, which is Stage 4, theta waves completely disappear, leaving only delta waves. Muscle relaxation is now complete. Pulse and breathing rates are the slowest, and blood pressure continues to drop during this stage. Stage 4 sleep—or delta sleep, as it is commonly referred to—is the deepest phase of sleep you experience. You are now in "never-never land" and are the most vulnerable to your external environment.

Delta sleep is the most restorative and healing phase of your slumbering process. Here the immune system is the most active and provides the highest level of infection-fighting capabilities. Since there are very few metabolic activities competing for your body's energy at this time, delta sleep provides the best opportunity for optimal tissue repair and cellular growth. The stimulation of this tissue repair and cellular growth is most affected by a very powerful hormone called human growth hormone. Human growth hormone is secreted by the anterior pituitary gland at various times of the day in varying amounts. However, it is secreted more during delta sleep than at any other time. This very powerful hormone is essential for muscle growth, body fat reduction and tissue healing. And get this, it is also the best known hormone for retarding the aging process.

But how can you elevate the secretion of this valuable "super-health" hormone? There are many natural ways to maximize the output of this valuable hormone while you sleep, as you will soon see. Even though this hormone is most abundant in teenagers, its production seems to commonly decrease with age. However, in athletic studies it was found that human growth hormone was maintained or even increased during delta sleep, despite the natural aging process, just by implementing a few healthy habits. The best-known methods for naturally increasing the output of this magical hormone during sleep are proper exercise, appropriate diet and the length and quality of sleep.

Regular exercise, specifically weight training, stimulates human growth hormone during sleep, probably better than anything you can do. Exercise as it relates to growth hormone and delta sleep will be discussed in more detail in Chapter 8. Correct diet is another very effective method for maximizing this valuable hormone. The particular diet that is most impressive in elevating growth hormone during Stage 4 sleep is, ironically, the one described and outlined in Chapter 6.

As you now know, a diet low in processed carbohydrates, moderate in protein, and adequate in healthy fats is the key to maintaining proper levels of insulin. And, believe it or not, higher levels of insulin in the blood, especially within a few hours of bedtime, inhibit the secretion of human growth hormone. There's that insulin word again! So, if you eat a meal right before bedtime, especially one containing processed carbohydrates, your anterior pituitary gland secretes less

growth hormone while you sleep. So, to maximize your human growth hormone production, avoid late-night snacking, especially the kind of snacks rich in processed carbohydrates. Better yet, bypass processed carbohydrate or starches altogether, and eat your evening meal at least two to three hours before your regular bedtime. You will feel the difference the
next morning—I guarantee it.

THE SLEEP CYCLES REPEAT

The first four stages of sleep from Stage 1 to delta sleep take around 90 minutes to complete, with delta sleep lasting between 30 and 40 minutes of that time. Once delta sleep ends, you start retracting back into the preceding stages--back to Stage 3, then to Stage 2, then to Stage 1. Interestingly, once you get back to Stage 1 sleep, you might think it is time to wake up. However, you are only beginning to sleep. Once your body retraces back to Stage 1 sleep, something very surprising begins to happen. Blood flow increases to the brain. Respiration, pulse and blood pressure elevate, and your eyes begin to dart back and forth.

This second passage through Stage 1 sleep is called REM, or rapid eye movement. Stage 1 REM sleep is very different from the initial Stage 1 sleep. Your brain is more active, your neuron activity increases, and your overall metabolic process picks up. At this point, you may experience your first dream. And believe it or not, everybody dreams every night. Even though you may dream in any of the four sleep stages, dreams occur predominately in this stage. REM sleep, like delta sleep, provides immense restorative powers. It has been said that delta sleep rejuvenates the body, while REM sleep restores the mind. REM sleep plays a significant role in facilitating storage, retention and organization of all information in your memory. It is also vitally important to your overall learning and cognitive performance.

Without the power of REM sleep, you would literally be lost mentally. The first REM sleep stage lasts from 10 to 20 minutes, with each recurring REM stage lasting longer.

After Stage 1 REM sleep, you proceed to Stage 2, then Stage 3, and then Delta sleep again. This second full cycle of sleep (REM, Stages 2 and 3, and delta) lasts from 90 to 100 minutes. These same cycles repeat until you awaken. Therefore, if you sleep eight to nine hours, you may complete six cycles of sleep. Studies have shown that the sixth cycle of sleep produces the longest REM stage, lasting up to 60 minutes. The longer you sleep, the longer you experience REM sleep. And the longer your REM sleep, the more health benefits you receive in terms of memory enhancement and peak mental performance.

WHAT ABOUT NAPS?

Naps are usually regarded as a lazy habit or unnecessary activity. However, some of the most influential and highly ambitious people in the world have been known to nap, such as Winston Churchill, Thomas Edison, John Kennedy and Albert Einstein. Even our former president, Bill Clinton, has been known to take a few afternoon snoozes. Outside our country, napping is much more accepted and commonplace, especially in warmer climates like Spain, Mexico, Central and South America and the Mediterranean region. But the good news is the acceptance of napping is slowly catching on as more of a productive activity than a waste of time. Even some businesses are trending toward specially designated times and places for short "on-the-job" snoozes in an effort to take advantage of the energizing effects of power napping. Research shows napping can be very beneficial, even if it is just for 10 to 15 minutes.

Now, how to nap. Noon to 3 P.M. is usually the best time to nap, since your body naturally takes a mental and physical energy dip during this time. This common afternoon energy lull usually corresponds to a slight body temperature drop. The duration of your nap is also very important. Generally speaking, a nap is most productive if it lasts from 10 to 30 minutes. If you recall, that is about the length of time it takes for the first two sleep stages to occur. If you nap any longer, you will enter Stage 3 or 4, which may affect your regular nightly sleeping pattern. You may also experience crankiness or grogginess by awakening in the middle of a deeper stage of sleep (like Stage 3 or 4). Nevertheless, just a short nap of 10 to 30 minutes can be enough to energize the mind and body for the remaining part of your day.

I learned another advantage of short afternoon naps from the training methods of Soviet bloc Olympic athletes in the late 1970s: It might interest you to know that the benefits of a power nap were certainly recognized by a brief but powerful output of human growth hormone. You may recall, growth hormone release is very instrumental in the body's repair process, muscle recuperation, body fat reduction and aging retardation. As part of their daily regimen, Soviet athletes scheduled regular nap intervals that noticeably improved workout productivity and maximized athletic performance. Maybe that's one reason the Soviet bloc countries were so successful in World Cup and Olympic competition. But don't think power naps are just for athletes. You, too, can benefit immensely from only a few minutes of afternoon shut-eye. This simple act can serve as a healthy boost to your energy and productivity and have a noticeable effect on your mental and physical health.

IN THE NEXT CHAPTER

Even though there are still many mysteries surrounding this dormant phase of our lives, one thing is for sure. Sleep does indeed affect our physical and mental health in many ways. But just how much sleep do you need? Are there ways to improve the quality of your sleep? Can you maximize the health benefits of sleep? Can our life span be affected by our sleep habits? These questions and more will be addressed in the next chapter. There you will learn how much sleep humans actually require and the best times to achieve quality sleep. I will also describe the ideal sleep environment and will recommend a proven and effective presleep ritual. See you in Chapter 8.

Chapter 8

SLEEP AND YOUR HEALTH

"Early to bed and early to rise makes a man healthy, wealthy, and wise."
BEN FRANKLIN

HOW LONG SHOULD HUMANS SLEEP?

That's the big question. We know now the average American sleeps less than seven hours a night. But how much is enough? How many hours do we really need? To hopefully shed more light on how long humans should sleep, I thought I would investigate some of our closest animal friends to see how long they slept. Maybe that would provide some clues. The investigation found some very interesting results. A donkey, for instance, gets about 3 hours of sleep; no wonder they're so dumb. A dog averages about 9 hours of sleep, although my dog seems to get a lot more. Man's closest genetic link, the chimpanzee, gets about 10 hours of sleep, as does the baboon. The fox and jaguar garner just under 11 hours. The gorilla gets about 12 hours of sleep. The wolf, raccoon and rat sleep around 13 hours. The cat slumbers for 15. And the flying mammal, the bat, sleeps nearly 20 hours a day. What an existence! But how long should you sleep? That's the question.

Dr. Peter Suedfeld of the University of British Columbia in Vancouver, Canada, decided to find out. He conducted a recent sleep study done above the Arctic circle that might give us an answer to this valuable question. This experiment was performed during the summer months in the North West Territories of Canada where the sun didn't set and daylight was constant. This was done to make sure that sunlight would have little effect on time judgment. Additionally, all other forms of time measurement were eliminated, such as watches, clocks and other timepieces.

A group of seven people were placed in this environment at a decommissioned weather station for the sole purpose of measuring sleep duration. Each person in the experiment was given a specific active daily routine with no particular time frame to complete. All work details and other activities, including meals and sleep, were left to the discretion of each individual. Every person recorded when they went to bed and when they awakened in a specialized activity log. This computerized journal kept track of their daily sleep duration without their being aware of it.

During the first couple of days, the group averaged a little over seven hours of sleep every 24-hour period. But as the experiment continued, each individual established his or her own unique sleeping pattern. Unaware of the time element, each person slept between 9 and 11 hours after the first week. In fact, by the end of the experiment the overall average sleep duration was 10.3 hours for each 24-hour period. Also, the participants took short naps in addition to the longer sleep periods more than 30 percent of the time. It appeared each person eventually migrated toward the sleep duration their bodies actually needed, and it would suggest that humans need closer to 10 hours of sleep a night instead of the recommended 8.

A much earlier study done by researcher Nathaniel Kleitman also confirms our need for more sleep. In this experiment, Kleitman and his colleagues wanted to see what would happen to human sleep patterns if all environmental time cues, including sunlight, electromagnetic forces and even cosmic rays, were totally eliminated. A test group was placed nearly a quarter of a mile deep inside a cave chamber located in Mammoth Cave, Kentucky, in order to avoid these particular time cues. The experiment showed that in the absence of time measurement, sunlight and geometric forces, the test group averaged nearly 9 hours of sleep for every 24-hour period.

However, researchers discovered an unexpected fact about the human sleep/wake cycle during this scientific experiment: As it turns out, these temporary cave occupants did not follow the expected 24-hour circadian cycle, which is consistent with earth's 24-hour rotational spin. Without the natural time cues like sunlight to orient them, the test subjects stayed up later and slept in longer, adhering to a 25 hour circadian cycle. Kleitman and his colleagues determined that the energy of the sun is what actually regulates our internal biological clock. Not only does this experiment suggest that humans need at least 9 hours of sleep per night, but it also demonstrates the importance of sunlight for maintaining our 24-hour biological clock.

What does the Kentucky cave experiment tell us? Well, for one thing, it shows humans do need more than the generally recommended eight hours of nightly sleep. And furthermore, it demonstrates how natural sunlight is the best method for adjusting our sleep/wake cycle. In fact, the most ideal activity you can do to set your biological clock is expose yourself to the sun's energy for at least one hour early in the day. (Exercise is also another method for helping to adjust the biological clock.) Keeping your biological clock set and maintaining a productive 24-hour sleep/wake cycle is very important for optimal human health. This means going to bed and arising at the same time daily, obtaining at least 8 hours of sleep per night and regular exposure to morning sunshine or natural light. This is very important information for those who have poor sleep habits or need help in waking up or going to sleep at a more desirable time.

Sleeping in on weekends to catch up on lost sleep during the week is not an effective way to achieve your sleep quota. This practice usually backfires by disrupting the sleep pattern, thus making it difficult to fall asleep at your normal bedtime on Sunday evening. Because of this self-created sleep cycle disruption, Sunday night is the most "insomniac" night of all. This is one of the main reasons that Monday is the least productive and the most "emotional hangover" workday of the week. If you must sleep in, make sure it's no longer than one hour, which usually doesn't affect your normal bedtime, provided you haven't napped excessively.

SLEEP AND YOUR HEALTH

The Arctic study and the Kentucky cave experiment substantiate the overwhelming data that adult humans need between 8 and 10 hours of sleep a night. Furthermore, scientific evidence suggests that the lack of quality, abundant sleep influences the strength and resilience of the body's immune system, which ultimately has a negative effect on our overall health. For example, an experiment conducted by Krueger and Toth involving test rabbits demonstrated how effective deep delta sleep is in repelling infection and serious disease. E. coli and other harmful bacteria strains were exposed to healthy rabbits over time while their brain wave activity was measured. In every case, the rabbits who experienced the highest amount of delta brain wave activity during sleep were the least likely to get sick. But get this—the rabbits with the smallest amount of delta wave activity during sleep not only experienced the most severe cases of illness but ended up dying as a result of the bacterial exposure. Clearly this shows how an organism's immune system and its ability to sustain life is greatly affected by the quality and length of deep sleep.

But what about human health? One particular study done at the University of British Columbia in Vancouver analyzed the data of 2,103 young adults to determine the relationship between length of sleep and the amount of visits to a physician. These healthy 18 to 25-year-old individuals were divided into three categories based on the amount of sleep they obtained. Participants who slept less than 7 hours a night were classified as short sleepers, while those who slept between 7 and 8.5 hours were called average sleepers. The ones who slept more that 8.5 hours a night were called long sleepers. Even though there was not enough meaningful data on the long sleepers to include them in the results, the findings do suggest a link between the amount of sleep and level of health, nonetheless. The results showed that during a one-year period the short sleepers averaged 3.7 visits to a medical doctor, while the average sleepers made 1.6 visits. In other words, those who slept less than 7 hours a night were more than twice as likely to become ill than those who slept between 7 and 8.5 hours. So, if you want to improve your health, get more sleep.

WHEN YOU SLEEP IS JUST AS IMPORTANT

Not only is getting enough sleep extremely crucial, but when you sleep is equally as important. The body operates on circadian rhythms, which are biological ebbs and flows taking place every 24 hours that correspond to the daily rotation of the earth. The body's sleep/wake cycle, hormone changes, enzyme production, fluid balance, and even body temperature are all connected to this 24-hour cycle. According to the latest research on biocircadian rhythms, there are daily energy fluctuations that take place during each 24-hour period that affect us all. These natural cycles or oscillations are influenced mostly by the sun's energy, time and gravitational pull. Case in point is the Kentucky cave experiment where the absence of environmental time cues altered the test group's 24-hour circadian cycle. These daily biological cycles are well founded in ancient medical and health practices called Ayurveda.

Ayurveda is the oldest known form of health studies that means literally "the science of life" and is based on five thousand years of Indian (from India) tradition and practical application. Just like the ocean's tides and the planet's rotation, the human body experiences daily circadian energy fluctuations that can be divided into six distinct time periods. According to Ayurveda, these times periods are 6 to 10, 10 to 2, and 2 to 6, and they repeat every twelve hours. Whether you know it or not, each person encounters different energy surges during these time periods. A good example of this is demonstrated by a mental or physical letdown many of us experience in the midafternoon (near the end of the 10 A.M. to 2 P.M. Ayurveda cycle). This is usually confirmed by a slight drop in body temperature. Another noticeable energy change is around 9:30 or 10 at night, near the end of another cycle. This usually corresponds to mental and physical tiring and a drop in body temperature as well. By staying awake past 10 P.M., you enter another Ayurveda energy cycle that usually contributes to a "second wind" or new-found energy.

According to Ayurveda research, the most pivotal time of day for regulating your energy rhythm and sleep cycle is 10 P.M. Staying up past, say, 10:30 in the evening places you into another Ayurveda cycle that usually energizes you, which may ultimately affect your sleep pattern. If you want to take advantage of these Ayurveda energy cycles, make a habit of going to bed by 10 P.M. Whether you believe in this ancient science or not, I can firmly attest to the validity of Ayurveda practices from the amazing health benefits enjoyed by many athletes and clients who follow it, including myself. That is why I stress not only obtaining a minimum of eight hours of sleep, but starting that eight hours as near to 10 P.M. as you can. Maybe it's true that early to bed and early to rise helps make a man healthy, wealthy and wise.

SLEEP AND LONGEVITY

Whatever your bedtime, the human body needs at least 8 hours of sleep; some need more, some need a lot more. Now, you may be able to function on less than 8 hours, but your margin of safety in terms of illness, disease and longevity is greatly reduced. That's right—even your life span is influenced by the amount of sleep you receive. Believe it or not, people who get more sleep live longer. In a six-year Finnish study tracking 10,778 adults, it was found that individuals who slept less than 7 1/2 hours a night, on average, were more than 2 1/2 times as likely to die during the test period when compared to the people who slept more than 7 1/2 hours. Likewise, the American Cancer Society conducted a much larger study following over one million volunteers for six years. It was concluded that people who slept the fewest amount of hours each night had the greatest risk of dying prematurely. Interesting, huh? So, if you want to add quality years to your life, make sure you get plenty of valuable, restful, restorative sleep.

SLEEP ENVIRONMENT

Improving your sleep environment is also another valuable suggestion for enriching the quality of your slumber. I suggest you use your bedroom for only two things; sleep and making love. Do not eat in bed. Do not argue. Do not start intense discussions that may lead to controversy, and do very little that might stimulate your mind prior to sleep. It is also not the time to start that crossword puzzle or balance your checkbook. Listening to light music, for example, is okay. Or even some light reading may be fine. But ideally you should develop the habit of using your bedroom for what it was designed, and that is sleep.

One very important no-no is watching television in your bedroom or, for that matter, several hours prior to sleep. The TV program content may arouse your nervous system, making it more difficult for you to reach the beneficial, restorative phases of sleep. Television viewing also stimulates the brain chemistry to produce more excitatory neurotransmitters like dopamine and norepinephrine, which suppress the deeper stages of sleep. There is also something about the TV screen and the energy it emits that stimulates beta wave activity and inhibits alpha wave formation. If you recall, optimum relaxation as well as Stage 1 sleep consist of alpha wave activity, and its hindrance will affect the initial quality of your sleep. Even though television and video screens definitely affect the brain and our sleep patterns, the degree of their disturbance is not yet completely known. More research is certainly needed in this area.

You may remember a few years ago in Japan where hundreds of youngsters all experienced convulsions or fits while watching the same children's television show. Apparently these simultaneous seizures were induced by the broadcast of a particular screen pattern and color scheme. Fortunately no one was seriously hurt during this bizarre phenomenon, even though many children had to be hospitalized. It just goes to show you the powerful influences television and video screens have on our brains. So, if you want to create a more sedate and relaxed bedtime atmosphere, avoid watching television at least one hour prior to sleep. This should be sufficient time for your brain waves to slow and mind to relax. Better yet, avoid evening TV viewing altogether.

The room temperature and humidity of your bedroom is also very important. Research shows the ideal temperature for quality sleep is between 65 and 68 degrees Fahrenheit, with a recommended humidity of 30 to 50 percent. A cooler sleep environment is much more conducive to lowering the body temperature and slowing metabolism, which is necessary to achieve a more dormant physical state. A higher humidity is most beneficial in minimizing the drying or dehydration of the delicate air passageways of the respiratory system. Since the humidity in most homes especially in the winter months is less than 15 percent, a room humidifier may be helpful. One of the real pleasures of my life is traveling back to North Carolina to visit my father and stepmother who are both in their eighties. The one thing I learned about bedroom temperature from personal experience is it's impossible to sleep in a room that is over 80 degrees. But that's another story. Since older adults may have poorer blood circulation and a less healthy metabolism, they need a warmer sleeping environment.

PRESLEEP ROUTINE

To help you develop a consistent nightly bedtime and maximize your sleep, you need to adopt a successful presleep routine or pattern. If you want to be in bed by 10 P.M., then start your nightly routine early enough to allow all the necessary activities to be completed. Such things as brushing your teeth, washing your face, showering and emptying your bladder are usually a part of most people's bedtime routine. But a truly successful presleep routine is more than just preparing your body for sleep. For effective, quality, deep sleep, you need to prepare your mind as well. In Chapter 12, I go into more detail about a very effective evening ritual that not only helps prepare you for sleep but can also help program your mind in a more positive way. For starters, I suggest you practice deep, diaphragmatic breathing that is described in Chapter 1. This helps create a more relaxed and peaceful mind and helps enhance a deeper, more restful sleep.

Another highly recommended presleep habit is the practice of complete silence. Every human being needs at least five minutes of total silence every day. This is best accomplished by sitting quietly in a private area and remaining as still as possible. Try not to think about anything as you close your eyes and relax. You may want to visualize a very peaceful and tranquil picture in your mind, one that is soothing and undisturbed. This type of visualization will help your sleep pattern and definitely promote a more positive frame of mind. You can practice this silence anytime during the day for that matter, but scheduling it just before bedtime will serve as a greater aid toward successful, restful sleep. One to five minutes of complete silence will help you be more receptive for the most important presleep habit of all. And that is prayer or meditation.

The practice of prayer or meditation right before you go to bed is probably the single most effective habit for ensuring a more restful night's sleep. Some people complain of not having a good night's rest due to anxiety or tension. Maybe it's worrying about a business meeting or an upcoming trip or some other apprehension that adds just enough stress to disrupt your sleep. Indeed, using prayer or meditation to communicate to a higher power about your worries and problems is the best antidote for minimizing a stressful mind before sleep. This could be applied to any time of the day, for that matter, but just before sleep seems to have a more profound effect.

One of the main reasons people do not get the quality sleep they desire is they usually carry an earful of worry and trouble to bed with them. If stress is one of your nighttime problems, let me suggest a Bible passage: "Let Him have all your worries and cares, for He is always thinking about you and watching everything that concerns you."This is one of my favorite verses, and I have successfully used it many times to squelch stress and other negative emotions and thoughts. Repeating this one verse in your prayers is one of the best methods for assuring you a more peaceful and restful night.

SUMMARY

As a recap, I would like to remind you of a few helpful suggestions for ensuring quality sleep. First, wake up and go to bed at the same time every day, including weekends. Second, properly prepare your bedroom environment. Activities like television viewing, controversial discussions, mental excitement and exercise (except sex) are likely to create untimely stimulation and should be avoided prior to bedtime. Refrain from consuming food or drink (especially alcohol) within a few hours of your normal bedtime. And most importantly, develop your own presleep routine (see Chapter 12 for more details) that involves deep, diaphragmatic breathing, silence, visualization and above all, PRAYER.

HEALTH HABIT 5:
Wake up and go to sleep at the same time every day, and achieve at least eight hours of sleep every 24 hours, weekends included. Even if you stay up later than usual, always awaken at the same time. Abstain from food or drink for two to three hours prior to your normal bedtime.

SECTION IV

EXERCISE

"Exercise is nature's self-appointed 'health optimizer.' It is the handicapper for our less than perfect lifestyle choices. It truly is the fountain of youth."

SAM VARNER, CSCS

Chapter 9

EXERCISE: THE REAL FOUNTAIN OF YOUTH

"If you could rank all the proven methods known to retard the aging process and enrich our health, exercise would be at the top of the list."

SAM VARNER, CSCS

Several centuries ago the famous explorer Ponce de Leon had a lifelong determination to find the proverbial fountain of youth. In every newly discovered land, he dreamed of finding a special water source or mysterious well that contained an elixir for keeping people young. Even though Ponce de Leon never discovered any fountain of youth, it still remains a passionate quest for many people, especially today. The pills, potions and cosmetics in our billion-dollar health industry are evidence of our society's continued fixation on everlasting youth and beauty. But if you could rank all the proven methods known to retard the aging process and enrich our health, exercise would be at the top of the list. It truly is the fountain of youth.

Exercise is nature's self-appointed "health optimizer." It is the handicapper for our less-than-perfect lifestyle choices. It can help level the playing field by overriding many of the negative consequences related to poor eating habits, overindulgent practices, stressful living and unhealthy addictions. Believe it or not, a recent study shows regular exercisers who smoke cigarettes have fewer health risks than sedentary individuals who do not smoke. As bad as smoking is, regular exercise can often delay many of the ill effects brought on by this compromising habit.

In another study, 40,000 postmenopausal women were observed over a seven-year period, and it was found that those who did regular exercise were 20 percent less likely to die prematurely than those who were sedentary. Furthermore, sedentary individuals are 80 percent more likely to develop coronary heart disease than more physically active individuals. In other words, of all the negative lifestyle practices that influence your health, the lack of regular exercise can have the most profound effect.

However, statistics show that most Americans are not sold on the need for regular physical activity. In fact, just last year the Center for Disease Control in Atlanta released an alarming statistic stating that over 66 percent of Americans do not exercise enough. Furthermore, 42 percent of the adults in this country are completely sedentary. The long-term effects of a sedentary lifestyle can have devastating consequences on your health in terms of quality of life, disease and even premature death.

In fact, your lifestyle may have more of an impact on your longevity than genetics. Scientists in Finland tracked the health and physical activity of 16,000 twins for 19 years and found that the twin who exercised at least 30 minutes six times a month, on average, was 56 percent more likely to have outlived his or her sedentary twin. The study also showed even sporadic exercisers tended to outlast their idle twins. Even though statistics show that most people haven't bought into the regular exercise habit, it should not undervalue the need for this disease-reducing, life-enhancing activity.

THE NEED FOR PHYSICAL ACTIVITY

Looking at the bigger picture, it is quite evident that the human body was constructed to move. Like all other animals, it is a movement organism. The human body is designed to walk, run, hoist, climb and do all sorts of valuable life-sustaining activities. If you were to study the structure of the body more closely, you would find the muscles, bones and joints all designed in a marvelous yet intricate balance. Each opposing muscle group is meticulously designed to move by pulling the skeletal bones they are attached to. The muscle-to-bone attachment (with the help of the tendons) creates a type of functioning lever that dictates a specific bodily movement. If you could see an actual dissection of the human hand or foot, you would be astonished at the elaborate construction of muscles, ligaments, tendons and bones all organized neatly as a functioning unit. And this impressive functioning unit is contrived to move. There are 630 muscles and 206 bones in the adult human body, with locomotion being their primary function.

However, one of the biggest drawbacks to our technologically advanced society, especially during the last century, is that we've drastically reduced the need for natural locomotion and physical output. We rely on the automobile, elevator, escalator and many other modern-day inventions that minimize our need to move and be active. Our lifestyle no longer revolves around hunting, farming and physical labor, and our 21st-century occupation is more likely to be sedentary than active. When the 20th Century came to a close, our top leisure time was allocated to television viewing, Internet surfing and video game playing. Unless you voluntarily create the kind of physical activity your body was designed to do, chances are your job or lifestyle won't be enough. Regular daily physical activity in the form of exercise is the only way to facilitate what your body was truly created to do.

WHAT DOES EXERCISE DO?

Regular exercise helps you look and feel better. It improves your health and reduces negative stress. It also heightens your energy level, while enriching the quality of your sleep. Exercise helps control your appetite and improves your thirst mechanism. It sharpens your mental concentration and enhances your memory. It also boosts your immune system and raises your tolerance to pain. Exercise incorporates deep breathing and involves muscular contraction, both of which activate a more forceful lymphatic flow. Exercise increases the body's sensitivity to insulin, while helping control blood sugar levels. And, exercise is the very best method for strengthening your heart, trimming body fat and sculpturing lean muscle.

Exercise does in fact produce a multitude of health benefits that carry over into many of the other principles in this book, and it is indeed nature's prescription for maximizing one's health. If you could put all the qualities and benefits of exercise into a pill and market it, you would actually have more than the fountain of youth; you would have the ultimate panacea of life.

EXERCISE REDUCES CHANCES OF DISEASE

Heart disease is the number one killer in our country today, with coronary artery disease and hardening of the arteries (arteriosclerosis) being the most common types. The risk factors for this dreaded affliction are hypertension (greater than 140 systolic and 90 diastolic blood pressure), elevated cholesterol (greater than 200 points), raised triglycerides (greater than 300 points), obesity and heredity. Even though you cannot choose your parents, you can dramatically reduce all other risk factors that predispose you to this degenerative illness simply by developing the exercise habit.

Merely one-half hour of moderate-intensity physical activity every other day has been shown to lower your risk of heart disease by as much as 60 to 75 percent, according to a published article in a recent issue of *Prevention Magazine*. There is no drug, medical treatment or modern-day therapy that naturally cuts the risk of heart disease like the magical habit of regular exercise. If only half of our country's nearly 115 million sedentary individuals walked just 30 minutes a day, this epidemic would be slashed by more than 50 percent. It would also be eliminated as our nation's top killer of adults. You have much more control over reducing your chances of getting this terrible disease than you might think, and it doesn't require that much effort either. So, for goodness sake, make your heart happy—take a walk!

The second leading killer in America today behind heart disease is cancer, which now afflicts one in two men and one in three women. However, statistics show only one in seven individuals who regularly exercise will get some form of cancer during their lifetime. Although there are many theories on the causes of cancer, its initial onset is attributed to one microscopic shortcoming—the lack of available oxygen on a cellular level. In the absence of this essential nutrient most cells simply die. However, not all cells suffer the same fate in a diminished oxygen environment.

Instead of dying, certain oxygen-deprived cells go haywire in their replication, resulting in abnormal cell growth. And if this bizarre type of cellular proliferation is not arrested by your body's immune system, these out-of-control cells become cancerous and oftentimes deadly. On the other hand, regular physical activity literally bathes your cells in this most indispensable nutrient. And it is this natural stimulation of increasing circulating oxygen to all cells that plays a major role in cancer prevention.

Frequent physical activity not only improves the circulation of oxygen-rich blood and other valuable nutrients throughout the body, but it also increases viable avenues for their transport. For example, regular exercisers have some 30,000 to 60,000 more miles of capillary blood vessels throughout their body compared to the average couch potato. Yes, that's right—30,000 to 60,000 more miles! Exercise stimulates the growth of additional passageways, which means more precious oxygen-rich nutrients are available for cellular support and nourishment. Not only does regular exercise increase circulating oxygen within the bloodstream, but it also establishes an additional network for its delivery.

EXERCISE AND THE LYMPHATIC SYSTEM

Physical activity is the result of muscular contractions. And it is these muscular contractions that directly stimulate the function of the lymphatic system. Remember how deep, diaphragmatic breathing increases the circulation of lymph fluid throughout the body and how this flow affects the rate of cellular waste removal. Well, exercise is just as effective at stimulating this flow. In fact, normal lymph flow is around 125 ml per hour. But moderate physical activity such as a brisk walk, invigorating jog, or light weight lifting workout increases the circulating lymph to over 1800 ml per hour. A more forceful lymph flow, as you recall, supports greater cellular waste removal and intensifies the formation of bug-fighting lymphocytes. So, just by getting your butt moving, you maximize your lymphatic system's ability to cleanse your cells and improve your immune system. It's no wonder your cells thrive on exercise.

EXERCISE IMPROVES THIRST SENSITIVITY

The daily habit of exercise stimulates your thirst for vital liquids. And it is this appropriate stimulation that enables your body to remain properly hydrated. However, unlike all other animals, human are not in tune with their true thirst sensitivity, which was described in Chapter 4. But regular daily exercise stimulates the effectiveness of your hypothalamus, which is the gland most responsible for stimulating your water craving. Even though exercise increases the need for hydration, it also sensitizes your thirst mechanism, which makes you more aware of your water requirement. Thus, you're more likely to drink more fluids.

EXERCISE AND APPETITE

How do you usually feel immediately after an invigorating workout? You're probably not ready to eat a big meal or munch on a snack. That's because your appetite is affected by the chemical and metabolic changes resulting from exercise. Even your craving for sugar-rich foods is diminished by exercise. One reason for this appetite suppression is the increased blood flow allowing more nutrients, especially oxygen, to circulate and satisfy your cells. Another reason is extra glucose being released from the liver into the bloodstream which stabilizes dwindling blood-sugar levels. This more balanced blood-sugar level increases the feeling of satiety, which eases food cravings.

But the most profound effect of exercise on appetite is the increase of a brain neurotransmitter called serotonin. Elevated brain serotonin levels help regulate your hunger and significantly suppress your craving for high-carbohydrate foods and alcohol. So, if you have a hankering for chocolate Kisses or bon-bons, go for a brisk walk, or do some jumping jacks. Your cravings will likely subside, and you'll trim some body fat in the meantime.

EXERCISE AND INSULIN

Regular exercise increases your body's sensitivity to the insulin hormone. Greater sensitivity to this potent hormone means your body needs less of it to respond to raised blood sugar levels. So, if a high-sugar meal or too many processed carbohydrates are consumed, a regular exerciser requires less insulin to stabilize the resulting spiked blood sugars. On the other hand, a sedentary individual who consumes a high-carbohydrate meal requires more insulin output to balance these sugars. And more insulin production, if you recall, is less beneficial for weight management, cholesterol control, blood pressure and overall health. In fact, just 30 minutes of mild exercise five days a week can positively affect the most powerful fat-storing hormone in your body—insulin.

EXERCISE, METABOLISM, AND FAT LOSS

Exercise increases your overall metabolism and improves your calorie-burning capability. This means a regular exerciser uses more energy and burns more body fat at rest than someone who doesn't exercise regularly. Just a short, brisk walk in the morning stimulates your body to utilize additional calories well after your walk has ended. Research shows a vigorous workout lasting around 30 minutes can activate your body's metabolism for up to 8 hours afterwards. For instance, if you ride a computerized stationary bike for, say, 30 minutes, you will probably burn around 200 to 300 calories, which may not seem like a lot. In fact, one Mrs. Field's cookie could wipe out all the calories burned during that bike ride. But the elevated calorie expenditure from that 30-minute session doesn't stop when you get off the bike. No, the calories continue to be burned like heat from the coals of a fire well after the blaze has died down.

Just think about it. If you exercise consistently, you will burn more fat even at rest than someone who doesn't. For example, let's compare two individuals who are physically very similar and who eat a comparable diet. The only exception is their exercise routine. One person exercises four days a week on average, and the other doesn't formally exercise at all. All other things being equal, the person who exercises regularly will burn anywhere from two to three times more calories during rest than the sedentary individual.

A regular exerciser also expends more calories while sleeping. This translates into burning more body fat during the least physically active time of the day. What a deal! You not only burn more fat during and after exercise but also while you sleep. Even less than ideal eating habits can be offset somewhat by a more effective fat-burning metabolism created by frequent exercise. Maybe this is one reason why people who workout consistently are less affected by dietary processed carbohydrates. So if you want to create a slender, better-sculptured body, a consistent exercise habit is a no-brainer.

EXERCISE IMPROVES YOUR MOOD AND EASES PAIN

Exercise is one of the best methods for reducing negative stress and easing mild depression. One reason is it stimulates the production of alpha brain waves, which facilitates a calmer, more easygoing disposition. Recall how deep, diaphragmatic breathing produces similar feelings of peace and relaxation as a result of alpha waves formation. Well, in terms of your mood, moderate physical activity works in much the same way.

Exercise also increases the level of brain serotonin which boost feelings of well-being, personal security, confidence and self-esteem. Higher levels of this mood-enhancing chemical increases your ability to relax and concentrate. Stop and think about it—don't you usually feel better after a good workout or moderate physical activity? Conversely, low levels of serotonin may increase your threshold to pain, contribute to fatigue and result in mild depression. If you have ever experienced anger, frustration or distress, a short bout of exercise may be all it takes to lift your spirits.

Besides altering your brain waves and elevating serotonin, exercise also stimulates the release of a special group of hormones called endorphins. Endorphins are natural euphoria-producing chemicals that elevate pleasure sensation and minimize pain. Simply put, endorphins make you feel good, naturally and safely. And isn't that what it's all about? In many cases, endorphin release is so exhilarating and invigorating it produces a kind of "high" that can be addictive—a healthy addiction. By sticking to a regular physical fitness regiment for at least six weeks, your body starts craving this exercise-induced "endorphin rush,"which helps ensure continuation of this very healthy habit.

When I used to work with stressed-out athletes or emotionally upset clients, one of my first suggestions to them to combat these feelings was to go for a walk or do some vigorous exercise. Not only did it take their mind off their problems, but it also produced some very positive chemical and emotional changes, changes that translate into a calmer, more improved disposition. I heard a great phrase while researching the information for this book: "A tired muscle is a relaxed muscle." It makes sense, doesn't it?

EXERCISE AFFECTS ARTHRITIS AND OSTEOPOROSIS

Not only does exercise help alleviate emotional distress, but it also eases the physical aches and pains associated with arthritis. Arthritis is a very painful and oftentimes crippling condition that affects over 18 million Americans. Even though it is thought of as an elderly affliction, many people in their fifties, forties and even thirties can experience one of the many forms of this joint disorder. However, more arthritis patients than ever are finding a great deal of pain relief when the proper amount of exercise, specifically weight training, is included in the rehabilitation process.

Up until a few years ago, it was generally thought that weight training for arthritics would put undesirable stress on the joints, thus worsening the condition. But recent medical findings now show that the proper type of physical activity does indeed decrease arthritis pain and improve overall healing. Mild stretching, light resistance exercises, walking and even aqua-training (exercise in the water) are activities that yield the greatest degree of relief from this debilitating disease. (Even additional quality sleep helps relieve some forms of mild arthritis pain.)

Regular exercise also lowers your chance of getting osteoporosis, which afflicts nearly 25 million Americans, mostly women and the elderly. Osteoporosis causes 1.5 million fractures in this country every year and costs $14 billion annually in medical bills and lost productivity. This disease results in an abnormal thinning of the bones, causing them to become weak and easily broken. There are measures you can take to help prevent bone loss, such as physical activity and adequate calcium (absorption) and vitamin D intake. Research shows that strength training and weight-bearing exercises like walking are the best activities for increasing bone density and reducing your chances of getting this bone-weakening disease. However, for those millions of Americans who already show symptoms of this ailment, proper exercise cannot only slow bone loss but can actually reverse the process in many cases.

EXERCISE SLOWS AGING

Exercise stimulates the release of additional human growth hormone (GH), which is the hormone most responsible for delaying the aging process and keeping you lean and vibrant. Teenagers naturally have the most abundant amount of this special hormone, but as you get older, you secrete less. However, certain lifestyle habits can affect the amount of growth hormone you release. The most important habit you can develop to positively affect your growth hormone production is regular exercise, no matter what your age. And weight lifting is the best form of exercise for increasing growth hormone output. Recent studies showed that elderly people, ages 75 to 90, who started a regimented weight-training program produced more circulating growth hormone than their sedentary counterparts. They also showed a marked increase in energy level, joint mobility, mental alertness and improved strength, proving that it is never too late to start an exercise program.

EXERCISE AFFECTS YOUR SLEEP

Exercise also helps improve the quality of your sleep. It facilitates a deeper, more effective Delta sleep phase, thus providing a much higher level of body restoration and repair. Research shows that Stage 3 and 4 sleep last several minutes longer and are more productive on the first and second night after a vigorous workout than on the nights following inactivity. These two phases of sleep are most beneficial for immune system buildup, tissue healing, cellular growth and body fat reduction. People who exercise, particularly those who weight train, fall asleep three to four times faster than sedentary individuals. Also, 30 to 40 minutes of basic weight lifting, for example, nearly triples the amount of human growth hormone released during Delta sleep for up to three nights following the workout. And having this much additional growth hormone makes a big difference in promoting a more restful night's sleep as well as delaying the aging process.

Exercise is also one of the best cures for jet lag. If you are traveling through more than two time zones, exercising on the day you arrive at your destination will greatly reduce the problems related to jet lag. When I traveled with the U.S. Ski team to Europe for World Cup events, the first thing our team did when we arrived was to workout briefly even though the previous night was spent on a plane traveling from the States. Just doing a light, sweat-breaking workout upon arriving at your destination makes a noticeable difference in rejuvenating the body and resetting your biological clock.

IN THE NEXT CHAPTER

Well, it's pretty apparent that regular exercise makes a big difference in the quality and health of your life. Being sold on regular physical activity, however, is only half the game. To reap its amazing benefits you need to take action, and in the next chapter I will describe the type of action you need to take in order to get the most out of your exercise habit. You will learn what exercises work best and what routines deliver the greatest health and anti-aging benefits. Whether you are an aspiring athlete or a 90-year-old great-grandmother, the information in Chapter 10 will point you in the right direction.

Chapter 10

THE EXERCISE LIFESTYLE

"Just do it."

NIKE COMMERCIAL

Hopefully by now, you are well aware of the tremendous physical, emotional and life-enhancing benefits of a regular exercise habit. Now I would like be more specific on the details of a daily exercise prescription that is best for you. For starters, I would like to classify an exercise program into two different categories. I call these exercise categories movement exercises and weight lifting exercises.

MOVEMENT EXERCISES

Movement exercises are activities that employ your body for movement or locomotion. The best examples of movement (aerobic) exercises are walking, jogging, hiking, swimming, dancing, biking and playing games like golf, racquet sports, softball and basketball. The reason I use the word movement instead of aerobic to classify this category is because aerobic usually insinuates checking your pulse, calculating exercise intensity, and staying within a certain heart rate range for a specific duration. The connotation of aerobic exercise is too formal and may be too intimidating to embrace.

In fact, science defines "aerobic" exercise as any activity that: (1) lasts at least 12 minutes without stopping, (2) gets you breathing deeply but not out of breath, (3) uses the muscles in the thighs and buttocks, and (4) keeps your pulse rate between 60 and 85 percent of your maximum heart rate. Now, mind you, you can follow the major guidelines for aerobic exercise if you're into that. But unless you're preparing for some specific athletic event or need to know your aerobic training zone, don't concern yourself with nomenclature. My goal here is to motivate you to do some form of active movement daily without worrying about following any cumbersome or confusing aerobic guidelines. The key to movement exercise is to get a little out of breath and have some fun doing so. Your goal is to just move!

A good guideline is to do some type of movement activity five to six days a week for a minimum of 30 minutes a day. And the 30 minutes doesn't have to be consecutive. You could take a brisk 15-minute walk in the morning and a leisurely 15-minute stroll after dinner to total your 30 minutes. And there are other productive but simple ways to add movement activities to your daily routine. If you play golf, don't take a cart. If you live close to your job, walk to work occasionally. Take the stairs instead of using the elevator whenever possible. Park your car as far away as you can at the mall or at work. Just by taking the stairs and parking farther away, you can log extra vital minutes of healthy exercise to your regular routine.

But more importantly you can scratch your name off the list of the nearly 115 million sedentary Americans there are today. A little bit of extra physical activity here and a little there done daily will surely make a difference in your overall health over time. The point is to physically move. Personally, I do some type of movement exercise every day but Sundays. As for you, I recommend being active and doing some form of physical activity five days a week, taking at least one day off. And having at least one day off will give you some deserved physical rest along with a well-needed mental break.

I am often asked what is the best exercise for losing weight and getting into better physical shape. My answer is the one you enjoy doing the most. If you enjoy jogging, then jog your heart out. If you hate to jog, then maybe walking is better suited for you. If you like neither, then find some activity that appeals to you. I have had some clients comment that they do not like any exercise—period. Some have even expressed a deep and passionate hatred for any form of exercise. I even had a very wealthy overweight client who hated exercise so much that he once said, "I can make a million dollars easier than I can lose weight." If you feel like you are in this category, then I suggest you closely read Chapter 11 on THOUGHT. As a matter of fact, making a million dollars and losing weight can be programmed in your subconscious mind in much the same way (but that's in the last chapter).

THE EXERCISE HABIT

Make exercise fun. One way to enjoy the exercise habit is to make it social. Join an aerobics class with your friends or get involved with a regular mall-walking group. Making exercise social can have a big impact on your consistency. One of the best and most effective exercise motivators is getting a workout partner with similar fitness goals as you. Finding a friend or neighbor to workout with on a regular basis will help you stay motivated and keep you more committed to a regular daily exercise routine. Music is another great exercise enhancer. If you ride a stationary bike or walk or jog, use music as a motivator. The rhythmic beat of stimulating tunes will help you overcome boredom and minimize physical discomfort as well as inspire you.

There are a lot of people who start an exercise program with the greatest of intentions but fall short of making exercise a lifelong habit. One of the main deterrents to continuing an exercise program is the lack of timely progress and a shortage of patience. Let's say you started a regular, daily walking program and were religious in your efforts. After four weeks of vigilant exercise, you see a minuscule reduction in your body weight. What would you do? You could either stay committed or get discouraged and give up. For many people, the discouragement of not feeling like they have accomplished enough in a certain amount of time is all the reason needed to quit exercising. Not seeing positive results in your exercise efforts is probably the number one saboteur to any workout plan. So, look at regular exercise as a means and not an end to your goals. Besides, nothing worthwhile in life was ever accomplished overnight. Be patient, make the process enjoyable, and I guarantee your regular efforts will pay off in the long run.

Another deterrent to the exercise habit is trying to accomplish too much, too often and in too little time, which almost always contributes to overtraining. Overtraining happens when not enough recovery time has allowed the exercised body to properly and efficiently heal. Some rationalize if a little exercise is good, then a lot must be great. This is what I call the "more is better" syndrome. But get this—the number one problem I encountered in training professional and collegiate athletes is overtraining. Yes, that's right. In my 25 years of coaching and personal training, I found overtraining to be the biggest detriment to an athlete's or client's physical progress. When you workout too much and too often, you set yourself up for increased fatigue, decreased motivation, increased chance of injury, heightened exposure to illness, needless muscular soreness and stagnating progress. All of this ultimately gives rise to discouragement and exercise burnout.

I have stressed doing some type of fun, exciting exercise for a minimum of 30 minutes daily, even if it's just a leisurely stroll. During a recent health clinic, I was asked the question, "What if I don't have enough time to get a complete 30-minute workout in. Do I just forget about it?"A lot of times, people are faced with a longer workout than they have time for. Instead of doing just part of the planned exercise routine, it is easier to blow it off, thinking such a short workout will do no good. This is how many individuals set themselves up to fail at the exercise habit before they even start. As I said earlier, it is better to break up your workout time than not to do it at all. Even it you don't have 30 minutes, then do 20 minutes, or 15 minutes, or even a 10-minute workout. The important point is to develop the habit of doing some physical activity daily.

Exercise doesn't have to be so formal that you monitor every workout with exact durations, intensities and heart rate checks, as some physiologists recommend, even though it's a good idea. Take a lean, healthy dog, for instance. A dog doesn't follow a specific aerobic routine or use any special devices like a pulse meter to successfully stay in shape. No, they just sprint a little, sniff around a little, run some more, lay down, get up, jump, fetch and chase. I think too many people try to split hairs and attempt to analyze everything scientifically when the bottom line is just move your body. The Nike commercials sum it up best by saying, "Just do it."And I say, "Just do something."

A lot of people tell me they can't find the time to exercise. I can appreciate that. But if you are waiting for extra time to fit it into your schedule, you will never develop the exercise habit. You have to make time. Schedule it in and prioritize it like any other important activity. If you don't make time to care for your body now, then your body will eventually rob you with less life at the end of your years. Optimum health is so dependent on the exercise habit.

I remember a story my college roommate told me that has helped with my time management even to this very day. He was majoring in premedicine and also playing on the college football team. The workload for school got so tough he decided there wasn't enough time for football. So when he discussed quitting the team with his coach, the coach told him something I will never forget. He told my roommate there are only 24 hours in a day, and everyone has the same 24 hours. The difference is how you use them. Now those are words of wisdom even time-conscious Ben Franklin would be proud of. By the way, those profound words were spoken by the famous football coach Lou Holtz. How are you going to use your 24 hours?

WEIGHT LIFTING

The second exercise category is called weight lifting and is probably the least appreciated and most neglected form of physical activity. Lifting or resistance training involves moving objects against gravity in an organized manner and is one of the most versatile of all exercise activities. It is used for a variety of purposes such as increasing strength, improving looks, losing fat, gaining muscle and rehabilitating injuries. Even though this healthy activity is usually accomplished in a gym or spa, you don't necessarily have to belong to a club to reap its amazing benefits. This is good news, since weight training in a public environment can be very intimidating for a lot of people. For those who dislike health clubs or find visiting them inconvenient, I will show you some very effective alternatives. But no matter where you lift weights or how you accomplish it, the most important objective of this exercise category is to hoist, tote, heft or lift against resistance.

The first known weight training or resistance exercise was documented during the Roman Empire and was used to help condition the powerful Roman soldier in preparation for battle. This particular strength-building exercise was called the dip and is similar to today's version of the ordinary pushup. The Roman dip exercise is where the body moves against gravity, using its own weight as resistance without the aid of any special equipment. (Gee, I wonder if they had conditioning coaches back then?)

The most common forms of weight lifting utilize barbells, dumbbells, selectorized machines and body weight exercises. Even hoisting heavy garbage cans or carrying grocery bags up the stairs can actually be a form of weight lifting. Resistance training, when done correctly and consistently, can produce some of the most remarkable cosmetic and health benefits possible. This may sound like a bold statement, but in all my years as a strength coach and personal trainer, I have witnessed firsthand the incredible benefits of weight training.

Athletes and nonathletes, young and old, males and females—all have excelled in this awesome body-building activity. Weight lifting is not reserved for the athletic he-man anymore, as housewives, elderly, and even disabled individuals all are pumping iron in much greater numbers. Whether you are a fierce Olympic competitor or a 70-year-old slightly overweight grandmother, weight training is an extremely valuable tool for helping you improve your health and reach your physical potential. And as an added bonus, a consistent weight-training regimen can do wonders for the emotional aspect by boosting self-esteem and overall confidence.

WEIGHT TRAINING IS FOR EVERYONE

But weight training hasn't always been the chosen form of exercise for maximizing performance and improving health. 23 years ago, when I started my strength coaching career, lifting weights for most sport athletes was frowned upon except for football players and a few other strength athletes. Many coaches thought the use of barbells would make an athlete slower, less flexible and hinder sports performance. Even though weight training has made tremendous inroads in earning its way to the forefront of enhancing performance, the general population, for the most part, has been slow to catch on.

One of the reasons weight training has taken so long to be socially accepted is due to many unfounded beliefs and widespread misconceptions. It was once thought that weight lifting didn't provide the benefits like those of aerobic exercise, such as improved heart and lungs, decreased body fat and lower blood pressure. Furthermore, it was even viewed by many as counterproductive to good health, causing higher blood pressure, elevated cholesterol and worn-out joints. However, current wisdom is now taking a more serious look at this activity as an equally viable method for improving overall health and well-being. In fact, the latest research now shows that proper weight training is just as beneficial and effective for improving your heart, lungs and circulatory system as aerobic exercise.

THE BEST WEIGHT TRAINING EXERCISE

A proper weight training program must consist of the right movements done correctly and in the appropriate sequence. The movement that is considered the best and most effective is the squatting motion. And the most basic exercise that involves this movement is called the SQUAT. For the experienced or physically able lifter, the SQUAT exercise is a knee bend movement or squatting action usually done with a weighted barbell on your shoulders or dumbbells held in your hands for added resistance. Advanced weight lifters call this movement the power squat, which is probably the most intense, most strenuous, yet most productive weight-training exercise you can do. For this reason, the power squat is known as the king of all weight lifts. For the beginner or physically less advantaged weight lifter, the squat exercise can be accomplished by doing a knee bend (it doesn't have to be deep to be beneficial) or a "sit down and stand up" motion.

The "sit down and stand up" exercise is usually the first weight-training movement I prescribe to my clients who are novice lifters, elderly or physically challenged. If you have never done this exercise or type of movement, it may sound a bit too easy—until you do it a few times. Right now, simply stand up and sit down in your chair 10 times without stopping, and see how you feel. Go ahead try it. It'll really work you. Once you get good at standing up and sitting down, place your hands out in front without using them for any chair or bench support. Doing this forces you to balance your body, working your hips and legs more thoroughly. Use your own body weight initially until you become more proficient with this movement. Then slowly add resistance either by grasping dumbbells or placing weight on your shoulders. Now you're doing the SQUAT. I cannot stress how important this squatting motion is for burning body fat, stimulating and sculpturing lean muscle mass, enhancing circulatory and respiratory function, and contributing to overall health.

But what makes this exercise so valuable? For one thing, it is the balancing of the weight (either barbell or body weight) and the type of spatial (where you are in space) movement that contributes to the success of this important lift. Also, this movement involves over 65 percent of all the muscles in your body, making it very effective and extremely time efficient. But the best merit of this exercise is it stimulates human growth hormone production more than any other exercise you can do. Remember human growth hormone? This is the hormone described in Chapter 5 that is most responsible for burning body fat, building strength, repairing cellular damage and keeping you youthful.

The squat is a compound exercise, meaning it involves two or more skeletal joints. In this case, the knee and hip are the joints involved. A compound exercise results in more growth hormone production, increases exercise efficiency, and gives you more "bang for your buck" than a single-jointed exercise. For example, a weight-lifting routine consisting of a compound exercise can be more effective and take much less time to complete than a weight-lifting program containing twice the number of single-jointed exercises. Compound movements are also systemic in nature, meaning they affect areas of the body that are not directly involved in the exercise movement. For example, the SQUAT directly exercises the muscles in the hips and legs. However, studies show that this exercise stimulates muscle toning and fat reduction in the upper body as well as the lower body. In other words, the SQUAT influences the entire body, making it a systemic exercise.

A recent scientific study supports the physical effectiveness and systemic nature of the SQUAT exercise. Anatomical measurements were taken at specific points on the hips, thighs, shoulders, waist and biceps before and after the experiment. The barbell squat was performed three times a week and was the only exercise done during this six-week study. The results showed a surprising reduction in waist size, even though no dietary changes were made. Body fat also decreased in spite of the absence of aerobic exercise. Furthermore, the muscle mass in the biceps and shoulders increased without the help of any upper body exercises.

This study demonstrates the awesome fat-burning power and impressive systemic effects of the SQUAT exercise. Some call it magic, but I call it nature's way of maximizing practical and efficient movements to promote a leaner, stronger, healthier body. So, if you want to shape and sculpture your current physique, start by implementing a regular weight-training routine that incorporates this simple, basic compound movement.

MY MOST INSPIRATIONAL CLIENT

Even though weight training is the best method for improving body strength and enhancing physical appearance, it is also one of the best ways of thwarting the aging process. A case in point is 96-year-old Mitsuko Bannai. At 86 and in very poor health, Mitsuko had just moved to the United States from her native Japan to live with her son and his family. The long-distance relocation, along with a prior intestinal surgery, left her practically bedridden and barely able to walk. The best thing she had going for her was a great attitude and tremendous emotional family support. At her age and physical condition, most would have expected her to live out the remaining portion of her life in the typical convalescent fashion. But not Grandma Bannai, as most everyone affectionately called her.

She was persuaded by an understanding daughter-in-law to try a specialized geriatric exercise program, thinking it might energize and strengthen her weak and brittle body. Since I had successfully worked with other elderly clients, it was decided that Grandma would be my next challenge. I started training her slowly and deliberately with a few basic exercises like special stretches and easy squat movements. She diligently and eagerly stayed with the prescribed two-day-a-week program, while I carefully challenged her with new and exciting exercises. Believe it or not, putting on a pair of boxing gloves and sparring with a special hand pad became her favorite exercise, not to mention her trademark around the gym. After several months of light resistance training, passive stretching and "fun boxing," her physical abilities and overall health underwent a miraculous transformation.

It is now ten years since Grandma Bannai made her first visit to our personal training facility in Salt Lake City, and her progress is nothing less than remarkable. In fact, a local TV station did a news story on the exceptional improvements created by her unconventional, life-saving exercise habits. This marvelous story is a credit to what sound exercise and a positive attitude can do for anyone, no matter how old they are or what condition they're in. I am very happy to report that Grandma Bannai just celebrated her 96th birthday and is still pumping iron twice a week and walking almost every day. Happy Birthday, Grandma! You are truly an inspiration.

No matter what your age or current physical condition, proper weight training can make an enormous difference in your health and well-being. Current studies are showing very promising results for elderly and infirm individuals who take part in specialized weight- training routines. In fact, a geriatric study involving convalescent patients between the ages of 70 and 90 demonstrated a 7 percent increase in muscular strength development after participating in a specially designed two-month weight-training regimen. Yes, that's right, individuals well into their eighties are starting to discover the therapeutic advantages of strength training, proving it's never too late to exercise no matter how old you are or how old you think you are. So, get out of your rocking chair, cinch up the lifting belt, and let's pump some iron.

HOW TO CONSTRUCT YOUR LIFTING PROGRAM

Okay, it's time to learn how to develop your weight-lifting routine. An ideal weight-training program should include at least one compound movement from each of the four basic weight-lifting categories. These four basic lifting categories are:

1. Upper body pushing
2. Upper body pulling
3. Lower body compound movement (pulling and pushing)
4. Trunk or midsection

Your weekly weight-training routine should include at least one exercise from each of the four major categories. For example, an upper body pushing exercise might include the pushup, body dip, incline press or bench press. A pull-down, pull-up or rowing-type movement would be classified as an upper body pulling exercise. The best lower body compound movements are the squat, leg press, step-up and lunge. And lastly, no sound weight-lifting program would be without a trunk or midsection exercise like the abdominal crunch or back extension. The trunk region deserves special attention because it is the anatomical center of the body and the source of great power and energy.

Obviously, intermediate or advanced weight lifters may wish to incorporate additional exercises that focus on specific muscles or isolated body parts. And that's okay. But my goal here is to stress the importance of doing a minimum basic weight-training routine comprising each of the four lifting categories. No matter what your age or current physical condition, you can find at least one weight-training exercise in each category to start with. As you improve, feel free to incorporate more challenging exercises, while increasing the load or resistance along the way. But please consult your doctor, or at least seek professional advice from a qualified personal trainer before you start any exercise program. A certified personal trainer is well worth the expense and will definitely save you time, money and effort in the long run.

After you decide on the exercises, you then need to determine the sets and repetitions of each exercise. Before I continue, let's go over some weight-training terminology that will be helpful. Here are two terms you need to know when putting together your routine—sets and reps. How many times you lift a particular weight or do a specific movement is called a repetition, and a group of repetitions is called a set. For example, if you do 10 pushups and rest a minute or so, then do 10 more pushups before moving on to the next exercise, you have completed two sets of 10 repetitions of pushups. I recommend doing one to three sets of 8 to 20 repetitions for most exercises, generally speaking. Again, I encourage doing at least one exercise from each lifting category per week. Keep in mind, however, my suggestions are only general recommendations. You may chose to weight-train up to six days per week and do more exercises per workout than I suggest. And that's perfectly all right. Your individual workout plan will depend, for the most part, on your current level of fitness, age, goals and weight-lifting experience. To give you a better idea, I would like to show you examples of three different weight-lifting programs that correspond to three various skill levels:

PROGRAM I

(Elementary Level)

DAY 1 (rest one minute between exercises)

Leg Press	1 set of 12 repetitions
Lat Pulldown	1 set of 12 repetitions
Chest Press	1 set of 12 repetitions
Abdominal Crunch	1 set of 12 repetitions
Stretching	

DAY 2 (rest one minute between exercises)

Leg Press	1 set of 10 repetitions
Seated Row Machine	1 set of 10 repetitions
Shoulder Press Machine	1 set of 10 repetitions
Low-Back Machine	1 set of 10 repetitions
Stretching	

PROGRAM II

(Intermediate Level)

DAY 1 (rest one minute between sets)

Leg Press	3 sets of 12 repetitions
Lat Pulldown	3 sets of 12 repetitions
Chest Press	3 sets of 12 repetitions
Abdominal Crunch	3 sets of 12 repetitions
Stretching	

DAY 2 (rest one minute between sets)

Hack Squat Machine	3 sets of 10 repetitions
Dumbbell Incline Press	3 sets of 10 repetitions
Bentover Rows	3 sets of 10 repetitions
Back Extensions	3 sets of 10 repetitions
Stretching	

DAY 3 (rest one minute between sets)

Leg Press (closer foot stance)	3 sets of 10 repetitions
Seated Row Machine	3 sets of 10 repetitions
Bench Press	3 sets of 10 repetitions
Reverse Abdominal Crunches	3 sets of 10 repetitions
Stretching	

PROGRAM III

(Advanced Level)

DAY 1 (rest one minute between sets)

Power Squats	4 sets of 10 repetitions
Leg Curls	3 sets of 10 repetitions
Standing Calves	3 sets of 10 repetitions
Hanging Abdominal Rollups	3 sets of 10 repetitions
Stretching	

DAY 2 (rest one minute between sets)

Dumbbell Bench Press	3 sets of 10 repetitions
Pullups	3 sets of 10 repetitions
Standing Military Press	3 sets of 10 repetitions
Dips	3 sets of 10 repetitions
Biceps Curls	3 sets of 10 repetitions
Stretching	

DAY 3 (rest one minute between sets)

Exercise	Sets
Squats (close foot stance)	3 set of 10 repetitions
Leg Curls	3 set of 10 repetitions
Standing Calves	3 set of 10 repetitions
Roman Chair Rollups	3 set of 10 repetitions
Stretching	

DAY 4 (rest one minute between sets)

Exercise	Sets
Dumbbell Bench Press	3 sets of 8 repetitions
Weighted Pullups	3 sets of 8 repetitions
Standing Military Press	3 sets of 8 repetitions
Weighted Dips	3 sets of 8 repetitions
Biceps Curls	3 sets of 8 repetitions
Stretching	

MOTEL WORKOUTS

For the best results in weight training, I recommend the use of barbells, dumbbells and specialized weight-training machines that can be found in most health clubs, gyms and fitness facilities. Even home gyms and noncommercial exercise equipment can deliver similar quality results if properly and consistently utilized. However, the lack of available equipment or fitness club access need not discourage your weight-training plans. While traveling around the alpine countries with the U.S. Ski team, I found it very difficult to locate quality fitness facilities for the purpose of continuing our team's in-season strength program.

But rather than eliminate this important component of our conditioning program, I devised several elementary resistance routines involving creative body weight exercises. By using innovative movements with your own body weight, you can accomplish a very worthwhile workout even without the use of the most basic weight-lifting equipment. Since most of these body weight workouts usually occurred in motel rooms during our World Cup travels, the athletes nicknamed them"motel workouts."A typical body weight or motel workout would look like this:

PROGRAM IV (MOTEL WORKOUT)

Bodyweight Squats	3 sets of 15 to 20 repetitions

(similar to the stand up and sit down movement, only without a chair)

Pushups	3 sets of 10 to 15 repetitions
Abdominal Crunches	3 sets of 10 to 15 repetitions

PROGRAM V (MOTEL WORKOUT)

Step Ups (use chair or bench)	3 sets of 10 to 15 repetitions
Bench Dips	3 sets of 10 to 15 repetitions
Abdominal Hip-ups	3 sets of 10 to 15 repetitions

PROGRAM VI (MOTEL WORKOUT)

Lunges	3 sets of 10 to 15 repetitions
Cheater Pullups	3 sets of 10 to 15 repetitions
Full Crunches	3 sets of 10 to 15 repetitions

Of course, these exercises could be modified to suit a more or less advanced fitness level. For example, to make a pushup easier, simply do it with your knees contacting the floor instead of your feet. To make a pushup harder, just elevate your feet onto a bench or chair, making it an inverted pushup. You could also use supplemental accessories such as canned foods, water containers and rubber tubing, for example, to add resistance and create additional movements. Devising and implementing a motel workout can be quite fun and challenging and can definitely prove helpful in certain situations. So, never let the absence of weight training equipment deter you from completing a successful resistance workout.

Developing a successful motel workout routine with the U.S. Ski Team later proved very useful for many of the collegiate athletes I trained. When I coached at the University of Utah, some of our Mormon student-athletes would choose to go on a two-year church mission during their athletic careers. While serving on their mission, it wasn't feasible to join a health club or spend hours lifting weights. But by utilizing brief motel workout routines, our missionary athletes were better able to maintain at least some type of physical strength during their sport absence.

WEIGHT-LIFTING GUIDELINES

Even though I have given you examples of several fundamental weight-lifting programs based on different skill levels, it would be impossible to devise an individualized routine for you here. The planning and implementation of an exercise schedule is ultimately your responsibility. I merely want to give you some direction in developing a basic strategy and hopefully inspire you to make it a consistent part of your lifestyle. The key is to just do it; just do some form of resistance training even if it's only for a few minutes a week. You could do some body weight exercises in your own home, or you could join a local health club. You could hire a fitness specialist to devise a workout, or you could learn how to devise your own. You might even need a personal trainer or lifting partner to keep you motivated. Whatever gets you going, just remember that a regular weight-lifting habit is a lot easier than you think and the rewards are invaluable. The point is for you to find a weight-training routine that's right for you and make it happen.

There are a few other important points about weight lifting that need your attention. First of all, always warm up before starting a workout. Warming up literally means elevating the body's core temperature. This is best done by actively moving the body, such as jogging in place, jumping rope, riding a stationary bike or merely moving your limbs around to increase blood flow. Doing very light resistance on the first exercise is another way of warming up. It's also a great way of preparing for heavier, more challenging lifts on succeeding sets. Breaking a light sweat is the best indication your body is warmed and ready.

A point that may surprise you is that stretching is not warming up. That's right! Stretching and warming up are two different activities. Consequently, I do not recommend stretching before your workout unless you have warmed the body first. A good rule of thumb is never stretch a cold muscle. The best time to stretch is at the end of a workout when your body is limber and loose. By stretching after your workout rather than before, your muscles are much more pliable and less susceptible to injury and strain. Remember, always warm up before your workout and especially before you stretch.

How you breathe when you lift weights is another important point, since a proper breathing technique can make a big difference in your performance as well as to your safety. A correct breathing pattern takes advantage of the position of your diaphragm muscle, which affects your exertion capability. This in turn increases your strength output and maximizes your workout. On the other hand, a poor breathing pattern can affect intrathoracic pressure and create cerebral tension, which may lead to headache, dizziness and neck strain. I have known some people to even faint during a workout due to incorrect breathing.

The proper breathing technique during weight lifting can be summed up in one simple phrase. Exhale when you exert: the x's always go together. This means you should exhale when you exert against resistance. For example, when you push away from the floor in the pushup, exhale. Conversely, when you lower your body during this exercise, inhale. Remember to always exhale when you exert. And never hold your breath.

For beginners, lifting weights twice a week for 20 to 45 minutes is sufficient to increase strength and fitness levels. If, however, you are a veteran weight trainer or have more lofty fitness goals, then increase the frequency of your workouts up to four to six times per week. But regardless of your skill level or how many sessions you do, keep the workout length between 20 to 60 minutes. And remember to build your program around compound movements for the most efficient, time-effective workout.

Your weight-training routine doesn't have to be long, strenuous or very complicated to accomplish the major health benefits discussed in this chapter. Personally speaking, my lifting routine used to last 1 1/2to 2 hours a day, three to five days a week. However, by reducing the amount of workout time to less than 35 minutes a session, four days a week, I noticed greater exercise intensity, improved strength, lower body fat, sharper mental concentration and a more invigorating workout. To this day I find it is much easier and much more productive to consistently follow a shorter, more intense exercise routine rather than a longer, more drawn-out one. And isn't that the key?

One of the reasons shorter, more intense weight-training sessions are better is human growth hormone production. Studies show that blood levels of this powerful hormone peak after 35 to 45 minutes of intense exercise. Beyond 60 minutes however, blood levels of this hormone subside and are much less effective. In some cases, it may even be counterproductive to pump iron any longer than 60 minutes from a hormonal standpoint. So, for the optimum weight-training session, keep it short, challenging and consistent, and by all means, make it fun.

YOU CAN DO IT

Hopefully, the information in this chapter has helped you understand how important and how vital physical activity is for maximizing human health and optimizing your well-being. This phenomenal elixir called exercise is for all ages, all fitness levels and anyone needing an edge in the game of life. Weight training and aerobic exercise are not just for the Olympic athlete or the football player, but they are for the 90-year-old grandmother, the business executive, the arthritic patient, the overweight housewife and most importantly, YOU. If you could put all the qualities and attributes of exercise into a bottle, you would have much more than the fountain of youth that Ponce de Leon was searching for centuries ago.

The regular exercise habit can offset many of today's unhealthy practices, such as poor diet, inconsistent sleep habits, negative stress and even smoking. Exercise is indeed health's equalizer. It has been proven beyond a shadow of a doubt that regular physical activity can help you look better, feel better, live longer and increase the quality of your life. We all have the same 24 hours in a day, and the ones who make exercise a consistent habit are the ones who will live a considerably healthier, more fruitful existence. So, make it happen!

HEALTH HABIT 4:

Do some form of aerobic or movement exercise at least five days a week, striving for 30 minutes in duration. Movements such as walking, jogging, hiking, dancing, playing games, biking, swimming and walking your pet are just a few examples. Your goal is to break a sweat or at least get a little out of breath.

HEALTH HABIT 3:

Do 15 to 60 minutes of weight training or resistance exercises at least two times per week, following the guidelines in this chapter on constructing a weight-lifting program.

SECTION V

THOUGHT

"It is your thoughts that control your actions. It is your thoughts that control your attitude. It is your thoughts that control your health. And it is YOU who control your thoughts."

SAM VARNER, CSCS

Chapter 11

YOU BECOME WHAT YOU THINK ABOUT

"Sow a thought, reap an action; Sow an action, reap a habit; Sow a set of habits, reap a character; Sow a character and you reap your destiny."

ANONYMOUS

In the previous chapters I have presented many principles that have been scientifically proven to enhance the health and quality of your life. Most, if not all, suggested habits are really commonsense concepts. In fact, everyone whether it shows or not has an inner desire to become healthier and live a longer life. But if practicing healthy habits can really extend the quality of your life and guarantee a more joyous existence, then why doesn't everyone follow a healthy lifestyle? After all, simply eliminating bad, less desirable habits and following good healthy ones is all there is to it, right? Sadly enough, knowing what to do and actually fulfilling it are two different matters.

FOLLOW THROUGH ON HEALTH

You would have to be from Mars not to know the dangers of smoking, yet over 25 million Americans still take those daily life-choking puffs. The dangers of drinking alcohol in excess are known to all, but millions still overindulge. Overeating and obesity pose tremendous health risks for shortening your life and minimizing its quality, yet 40 percent of our population is classified as obese and nearly 60 percent are overweight. If the unhealthy practices of overeating, smoking and overconsumption of alcohol are so detrimental to one's health, then why do so many people continue to overindulge?

The key objective of this book is not the importance of learning all the health habits described or understanding how they work. Although that is very important. The fundamental objective is to help you make these healthy habits a consistent part of your daily routine. Even if you embrace every major point in the previous chapters, it will do you no good unless you implement these principles into your life. Just knowing that a habit is healthy for you is not enough. The knowledge is worthless and will not benefit you at all unless you take action. And that is the purpose of this chapter: to help you make these valuable principles a reality in your life.

I will show you how to successfully program your mind to generate any consistent pattern you desire such as a new health habit or worthwhile goal. If you want to get more quality sleep or eat fewer processed carbohydrates or follow through on your daily exercise program but can't seem to develop the habit, then this chapter is for you. If you want to know how to be healthier, you should study the principles in previous chapters, but if you aspire to effectively implement these daily habits into your life, then read on. I will show you how to establish a healthier lifestyle and stick with it. I will also show you how to overcome negative addictions and develop daily practices that foster lifelong health and success.

OWNER'S MANUAL TO THE MIND

What if you purchased a fancy, brand new computer and didn't receive the owner's manual? All you really knew about the computer was how to set it up, turn it on and what you observed others doing with their computers. To learn more about using the computer, you would experiment by punching different keys and seeing what each key function did to the screen. Even without knowing how to use your new computer, the pull-down windows along with the mouse would make it easier to improve your learning efficiency. You could even seek the assistance of a specialized tutor or enroll in a computer class to better your knowledge and use of this newly purchased hard drive. But quite frankly, you would by no means come close to tapping into the magnificent power of this awesome technological hardware without the help of the owner's manual.

Operating a computer system without the aid of an owner's manual closely parallels the use of our human mind. If you really stop and think about it, your mind came as standard equipment at birth without instructions. Learning how to use this incredible tool depended mostly on what you observed from your parents and your environment, just like learning to use the computer from watching others. Most computer experts agree that the average computer user employs less than 20 percent of its potential. The same can be said for the human mind. It's like we've been given this awesome computerlike brain but haven't fully learned how to use its amazing power. The sad truth is that most people never realize their mind's capabilities. So how can you raise the threshold of your mind's capacity without the so-called owner's manual? How can you tap into the incredible abilities within your powerful human computer? And if there was an owner's manual for the human mind what would it tell us?

YOUR COMPUTER MIND

It would tell us, ironically, that the human mind functions very much like the most powerful computer systems in the world. In fact, you process information and produce actions in much the same way a computer acquires information and performs tasks. Your mind collects information via your senses just like the computer receives data from its programmer. The subconscious mind absorbs the millions of bits of information from what you see, hear, feel, taste and smell and then stores it. And its how you assimilate and utilize this stored information that affects your actions and behavior. In effect, if you are to control and manage your behavior, then you must first learn how to control and manage your mind. And this can be achieved by programming the subconscious part of your mind. So, how do you program your subconscious mind? Is there some magical or scientific way to accomplish this?

YOU BECOME WHAT YOU THINK ABOUT

The answer is YES. Yes, you can program your subconscious mind, and yes, it is both magical and scientific. In fact, if there were a written owner's manual for your mind, it would contain just six simple words. This six-word operational guide is based on a very elementary law of nature that applies to every human being without exception. If you grasp this basic natural law, your life will be changed forever. Understanding these six words will better enable you to successfully program your all-powerful, computerlike mind. The six words are "You become what you think about."

In Earl Nightingale's best-selling motivational tape produced in 1956, his whole philosophy is based on this one simple premise. In fact, it's so remarkable yet so simple that most people aren't even aware of how their thoughts direct their lives. That's probably why he entitled this million-selling motivational hit, "Life's Strangest Secret." Strange because science doesn't fully understand how the human mind works, and the secret is most people haven't learned to harness its immense power. Achieving abundant health and success in life starts by learning how to manage the awesome machine between your ears. If you think success, you will achieve success in whatever endeavor you pursue. It's all in how you use your thoughts.

Every successful accomplishment was initially conceived from a simple thought. The house where you live, the furniture you are sitting in right now, and the car you drive was originally created in the form of an idea—an idea that sprouted from someone's mind. Just think about it—nothing manmade was ever created without a thought-producing idea. And it's the action taken from an idea or thought that produces the appropriate behavior. Even the most subtle thoughts elicit behavior, be it positive or negative. Those same powerful thoughts that produce positive human behavior can be a two-edge sword. It can direct a person to the top of the company ladder or into the gutter. It's all in how you use it. Both success and failure in any endeavor have their origins from the thoughts in your mind. It has been said, "We are the sum total of our thoughts." That's right—our thoughts, whether they are positive or negative, mold our behavior and subsequently our future. And being able to master or control your thoughts is the key to successful healthy living.

Sow a thought, reap an action. Sow an action, reap a habit.
Sow a set of habits, reap a character.
Sow a character and you reap your destiny.

MASTER YOUR MIND

There have been numerous studies done on the common traits of the most successful people in the world. From Plato to Lincoln, from Gandhi to Edison, they all had one thing in common: They became the masters of their thoughts. You see, I don't believe in luck, but I do subscribe to the philosophy that people subconsciously dictate their future whether they know it or not. Every thought, idea or perceived event that you have ever encountered is stored somewhere deep in your subconscious mind. Think about it. Whether you remember it or not, the perception of your first day of school is filed deep in your subconscious. That first kiss and how you felt lie tucked away in your mind's recesses and may or may not be recalled by the conscious mind.

Your mind truly is an amazing cognitive instrument that possesses the mysteries of an undiscovered frontier. Universities have proven we only use about 10 percent of our mind's capacity. I maintain that most people never fully utilize the magnificent power between their ears. But how can you tap into the power of the mind? Can you really design your future merely by controlling your mental cockpit? Why do some people become successful and other become failures as they go through life? Why do some avoid destructive habits like the plague, yet others embrace them? The answer lies in you. That's right—Your thoughts are the fuel of your mind's potential. Ralph Waldo Emerson wrote, "You are what you think about all day." Marcus Aurelius, the great Roman emperor once said, "A man's life is what his thoughts make of it." But Buddha conveyed it a little more forcefully: "All that we are is the result of what we have thought about. The mind is everything. What we think, we become." Believe or not, every person is where they are in life right now because that is where they really want to be, whether they know it or not. Sure, environmental and social factors affect your status, but your ability to control your thought process is the key to being able to rise above adverse situations.

Positive Thoughts
Create Positive Habits

The Bible says, "As you sow so shall you reap." What you plant in your mind with your ideas and thoughts will inevitably produce your actions. It's like your mind is a plot of rich, fertile soil. You, as the farmer of your mind, have a choice to plant whatever you want. For example, if you plant flower seeds a garden, water, nourish and care for them, they will produce a wonderful array of the most beautiful flowering plants you can imagine. But if you don't plant anything in your abundantly rich, garden soil, you may or may not produce flowers. But most assuredly your garden will yield many unsightly weeds. The weeds, if left unchecked, will eventually choke off any beautiful flowers that were lucky enough to grow.

Your mind is no different than the fertile soil in that garden. The thoughts you plant in your mind are the seeds of what you will eventually reap come harvest time. In fact, the mind is so fertile that even if you don't plant the seeds of successful thoughts, you will be vulnerable to whatever the winds blow into your mind's subconscious soil. In other words, your mind may be easily swayed by both positive as well as negative thought. And in most cases, the negative thoughts are so subtle you may not even be aware of their damaging presence.

THE POWER OF THE SUBCONSCIOUS MIND

I'll give you an example. I was in the grocery store the other day and noticed a mother scolding her child after he had accidentally knocked over a canned-food display. The mother shouted, "Just look you! Why are you always so clumsy? You're a naughty little boy!" Yes, the child did make the mistake of bumping over the display, but the mother's reaction of yelling negative, degrading comments was far more damaging. If you continue telling someone how bad or inept they are, they may start to believe it.

A mind will construct behavior to fit recurring mental images. And if the mind visualizes itself as being inept or bad, it will usually create behavior to fulfill that picture. Even if the conscious mind doesn't accept the negative comments, they are absorbed by the subconscious mind, possibly affecting future behavior. Children are especially impressionable to negative (or positive) comments that could last a lifetime. So, if you want to instill confidence and self-esteem in youngsters, you can begin by affirming positive statements that encourage successful behavior.

AFFIRMING POSITIVE THOUGHTS

Whether it's the growing mind of a little kid or a mature adult one, affirming positive thoughts enables the mind to construct successful behavior. Maintaining a positive attitude and minimizing negative thoughts require effort. It is easier for a person to think negatively than positively. That's why most people never achieve the success they really want. But how can one create an atmosphere of positive thinking while minimizing the negative impulses? Set yourself a conscious task. That is, once you notice a negative thought entering your mind, override it with an equally powerful positive thought. Painting a picture of the positive thought will better enable you to eliminate the unwanted negative thought.

A good example of this involves college basketball players and their foul-shooting abilities. At Utah, players were taught to picture themselves making successful free-throws over and over again in their minds. By repeatedly visualizing foul shots, success in live game situations was maximized. If an image of missing a foul shot ever came to mind, the players were taught to shrink the unwanted image while simultaneously enlarging the desirable picture. Think of it like a split-screen television where the shrinking negative image is replaced by an expanding positive one. The more you practice this mental picture swap, the more likely you are to affirm positive behavior.

Another example of the power of visualization involved the

training of U.S. Ski team athletes. It was demonstrated in an experiment that five hours of actual training on the slopes combined with one hour of visualization proved more effective than six hours of training alone. The more you practice visualization, the more likely you are to control the direction of your thoughts. And by mastering the quality of your thoughts, you guarantee a more positive pattern of behavior.

Mastering your thoughts also affects your attitude. William James, the great psychologist, once said, "The greatest discovery of my generation is that human beings can alter their lives by altering their attitudes of mind." Happy thoughts, sad thoughts, angry thoughts, they all are manufactured initially by what you plant in your mind. I firmly believe that most unhappiness is created by unhappy thoughts. Leading health experts agree that almost all illnesses and diseases have roots in undesirable emotions like hate, anger and stress. All of this stems from negative thinking.

Hippocrates once said, "The natural force within each one of us is the greatest healer of disease." Overcoming negative emotions is the first step in promoting a healthier, more harmonious life. And it all starts by learning to direct your thoughts. It has been said that you are either the master of your thoughts or a slave to them. Which are you? Are you going to let the winds blow just any seed of thought into your receptive, fertile mind, or are you going to control what you plant? Positive thinking or negative thinking—it's your decision.

THOUGHT QUESTIONS

But how does ones create an atmosphere of positive thinking? If just thinking positive thoughts is all it takes to be happy and successful, then why doesn't everyone achieve happiness and success? Positive thinking is more than just repeating affirmations or forcing yourself to think happy thoughts. You can chant success slogans or mantras all day long, but you probably won't create the desired positive thought process unless you learn to direct your subconscious mind. But how can you do that? Actually you can program your mind in much the same way you program a computer to solve problems: Input the problem in the form of a question. This commands the computer to search its data banks, process the information, and arrive at a solution.

Your mind, like the computer, works in much the same way. Your thoughts in the form of questions stimulates the mind to search its data bank and generate an answer. Even the simplest or most rhetorical question elicits a response. For example, a subtle thought like "Why can't I do this?" will produce a search for a solution. Questions like this are called presuppositions, meaning they presuppose the question to be true beforehand. The problem, however, is that negative presuppositions give your mind a foundation for negative thinking. And believe it or not, your mind will find reasons why you think you can't do something if that's what you think. No matter how trivial this might seem, your mind works on this level. So, if you ask negative questions, your mind will look for negative responses. Ask positive, thought-provoking questions, and your mind will look for positive, workable solutions. This is the first step to successfully programming your mind.

As a personal trainer, I saw this type of negative questioning undermine many people's efforts to lose body fat. Even simple little comments like "It's just too hard to lose weight" or "I guess I'm destined to be fat" will affirm your current overweight behavior and guarantee you'll stay there. Most unwanted behavior or undesirable habits originate from self-sabotaging subconscious impulses. And these subversive impulses are sowed by negative thoughts. For example, if someone has a difficult time trying to lose weight, they may pose the question "Why can't I lose weight?" Do you see how presupposingly negative this questions is? You end up blowing off workouts or eating the wrong foods and wonder why you can't lose weight. Your subconscious mind absorbs these negative questions like a computer assimilates data, and the end result is usually self-sabotaging behavior.

To take advantage of the immense potential of your subconscious mind, pose more empowering questions. Thought-questions like "What can I do to lose body fat?" or "How can I have fun getting into shape?" will foster more positive-directed impulses. As your mind searches it data bank, it will subconsciously arrive at productive, fun ways to lose weight. After my clients began practicing this type of mental questioning daily, they noticed a dramatic increase in the urge to exercise, avoid unhealthy foods and strive for better health. Therefore, to promote healthier behavior, ask the right thought-provoking questions daily upon arising and before retiring. Simply put, you have a choice—program your subconscious mind with positive empowering questions or with negative self-sabotaging ones. It will make a huge difference in your future-creating behavior.

PROPER GOAL SETTING

Even though affirming positive mental questions to yourself is an effective way of creating more desirable behavior, it is not the only way. Another equally important method for programming your subconscious mind involves the art of goal setting. Webster defines a "goal" as "an object of ambition or effort or a destination." Most people are acquainted with the idea of setting goals but fail to reap the astonishing benefits of proper goal setting. Simply making New Year's resolutions without following through is certainly not correct goal setting and usually produces less than successful results. Nearly 60 percent of Americans set New Year's resolutions, most of which are broken by the end of January. However, less than 2 percent of this country's population has written well-defined goals with a plan for their implementation. Surprising, huh? Oddly enough, people spend more time planning a vacation with the routes to take and places to stay than planning their life's future.

One of the most profound sociological studies conducted many decades ago really demonstrates the power and magic of goal setting. The 1953 graduating class of Yale University was evaluated on several aspects of life, business and future plans. In this in-dept study, it was determined that only 3 percent of the senior class had written well-defined goals. After two decades, the living members of this class were involved in a follow-up study to determine how the class had fared since graduation. According to the subjective evaluation, the 3 percent that had the written goals were happier, healthier and better adjusted in terms of business, social and personal aspects of life. Even though these results were subjective in nature, they signify the overwhelming importance of goal setting. However, the most objective evaluation of this study proved to be the most interesting. In terms of monetary success, the 3 percent who set written goals with a definite plan accumulated more financial wealth than the remaining 97 percent combined!

My point here is to stress the importance of writing and focusing on what you really want in life, not only in the area of physical health but in all aspects. When you write a definite plan for your future and focus on it daily, you are consciously transmitting thought energy to your subconscious mind. Remember, you become what you think about, and if you think about your goals in a relaxed, positive atmosphere, your mind begins to create behavior that subconsciously drives you toward your focused plan. There are unknown forces at work in life and throughout the universe that respond to the magical vibrations created by our thoughts. Focusing on your goals consistently is one of the most powerful tools for creating the future you desire in advance. And it is also the best way to define your destiny. Please do not take lightly the power of goal setting. With a purpose and faith, anything can be accomplished—I repeat, anything! So, in order to ensure a happier, healthier, more prosperous life, write your most important (health) goals and review them daily.

PURPOSE AND FAITH

The key to any goal is having a definite purpose. Your reasons for accomplishing any goal must be so compelling and so inspiring that you will stop at almost nothing to achieve it. This is the kind of relentless objective you need to ensure complete success. That is exactly why each health principle described throughout this book is accompanied with substantiated proof and compelling arguments. Once you have defined your goal and have an unequivocal purpose, simply blend in faith. Faith is the magic ingredient and is the driving force behind any successful accomplishment. Lack of faith is probably the number one saboteur of any aspiration. Sure, one needs persistence and hard work, but encountering too much resistance when working toward a goal will zap your faith quicker than anything. Here's my remedy for overcoming the shortage of faith.

The definition of faith is having complete confidence or total trust. And the best way to instill confidence in any endeavor is to have success in it beforehand. If you successfully complete a task repeatedly, your confidence in that task will soar. But what if you have never tried an activity, or worse, you attempted the activity and failed. How is it possible to gain confidence in situations like this? The answer is mental practice. Yes, practice the activity's positive completion in your mind over and over again. In other words, visualize the success in advance by seeing, feeling, hearing and "emotionalizing" every detail of your desired result. In fact, successful goal setting is not possible without this important art of visualization.

PRACTICE VISUALIZATION

Michael Jordan, the greatest basketball player of all time and future NBA Hall of Famer was once asked how lucky he must have felt to be blessed with so much talent and athletic ability. His reply was. "Athletic ability and talent will only get you so far, but it's desire and all the hours of practice that have enabled me to succeed with my God-given talent." Without polishing your talents with relentless practice, your abilities will not shine. And it's not only physical practice but also the mental practice that's important. I remember standing at the start-gate before World Cup ski races and observing many of the top skiers closing their eyes and gesturing their hands as if they were already successfully shushing down the race course. In the locker room before every football and basketball game, I would see many athletes momentarily close off the outside world just to picture their own successful game in advance. Like the athlete preparing for an event, the more you visualize, the better your chances of improving the outcome. So, if you want to maximize the power of your goals and boost your confidence, simply visualize reaching your desired target everyday, and your faith will blossom.

ESTABLISHING A HABIT

Once you understand the importance of goal setting, faith and the value of visualization, you are now ready to learn the fundamentals of creating habits. The dictionary defines "habit" as "a regular tendency or practice, an addiction, a mental constitution or attitude." It has been said that human beings are creatures of habit, regularly performing tasks or rituals sometimes without even consciously thinking about it. Take brushing your teeth, for instance. For most of you, this hygienic practice is such an ingrained habit that you don't even think about it—you just do it. I'll bet, however, that the habit of brushing your teeth didn't happen overnight. As a child, I'm sure your parents encouraged or even threatened you to perform this regular custom. Or maybe the intense pain of a few cavities from not following through swayed you to make it a consistent practice. Regardless of the reasons, establishing a daily habit like brushing your teeth requires a method, a method that's easier than you might think.

To successfully implement a habit and make it a consistent part of your lifestyle requires four fundamental steps. The first step is to decide to do it and make it your goal. You need to be 100 percent committed to your goal to ensure its success. Once you make the decision, write down your desired goal on a card or in your personal planner and review it daily. (see Health Habit 2). Secondly, focus on your goal often by thinking about it and asking positive, thought-provoking questions. That's right—ask thought questions about your goal. The third step is have a definite purpose for accomplishing your new goal. Take the time to write compelling reasons why you must create this habit, and be specific. And fourth, attach or associate intense emotions of pain and pleasure to the visual outcome of the habit you wish to adopt or change. After all, seeking pleasure and avoiding pain are the ultimate driving forces for human behavior.

So, if you wish to instill a healthy, desirable habit, first decide to do it by making it your goal and committing 100 percent to it successful outcome. Second, ask positive thought questions about your desired healthy habit. Third, what's your purpose or reason for following this habit? Write compelling reasons why you must establish this healthy habit. Finally, visualize an enormous amount of pain to not following through on this habit. How will you look, feel and be years from now if you do not practice this habit regularly? Emotionalize the pain; make it real.

After all, you already do this on a smaller scale, and you're probably not even aware of it. Let's use the habit of brushing your teeth again. Why do you do it? Well, whether you are aware of it or not, you link a certain degree of pain to not performing this daily ritual. That's right. I am sure that on some mental level, you have imagined the pain of tooth decay, bad breath, gum disease or yellow teeth, which is ultimately what drives this habit. In addition, you probably associate a certain amount of pleasure to a beautiful smile and clean-smelling breath. That is also a very compelling reason. However, in terms of human behavior, avoiding pain is usually a stronger motivator than seeking pleasure, so let's take advantage of that.

After you have visualized lots of pain to not installing this habit, now mentally associate a huge amount of pleasure to mastering it. You'll certainly be ready for this if you've effectively visualized enough pain. It is very important to emotionalize the pleasure you'll receive from accomplishing this goal. How will you look, feel or be months or even years from now if you master this habit? Again, make it real. The interesting aspect to this pain/pleasure mechanism is how your subconscious mind responds. Even though your conscious mind creates the pain/pleasure imagery, it is your subconscious mind that picks up these mental pictures and dictates your urges, hunches and ideas. And it is these urges, hunches and ideas that steer your actions, ultimately directing your behavior—a behavior that is more conducive to reaching your desired goal.

If you visualize enough pain to avoiding a habit and enough pleasure to implementing it, your mind will successfully adopt it. It usually doesn't happen overnight, and it may take some time, but it does work. Whether it's the simple habit of brushing your teeth or a much greater one like exercising regularly, the same concept applies. Even getting rid of an unwanted habit like smoking or eating too much can be achieved by following the same four steps. And the key to these fundamental steps is using the pain/pleasure mechanism. After all, your mind uses this emotional device all the time, so why not learn how to harness this power and use it to your advantage. So, if you want to establish any healthy practice, all you have to do is master the thoughts that control this important emotional mechanism.

THE POWER OF THOUGHTS

You can use the powerful thoughts of your mind to develop your future, a future full of health and prosperity. Expect the best and get the best; expect the worst and you will probably get the worst. Define your goals, study them regularly, visualize their achievement in your mind's eye, and blend in faith. Remember, faith is the magic ingredient. As William James once said, "Our belief at the beginning of a doubtful undertaking is the one thing that insures the successful outcome of any venture." And the great positive thinker, Norman Vincent Peale, said, "When you expect the best you release a magnetic force in your mind by a law of attraction. This force tends to bring the best to you." Not only does this help you establish desirable habits, but it is fundamentally how you achieve the successful life you truly deserve.

The main focus of this chapter is on THOUGHT and how it can direct human behavior. Writer James Allen was quoted as saying, "Clean thoughts make clean habits." It is indeed your thoughts that control your habits. It is also your thoughts that control your actions. It is your thoughts that control your attitude and ultimately your health. And it is you who control your thoughts. Good thoughts can never produce bad results, and bad thoughts can never produce good results. Thoughts are indeed dynamic energy vibrations that are like special radio waves being transmitted and received through a very powerful medium called the human mind. And it is how you focus this immense mental force that determines the quality and potency of these magical waves called thoughts.

Chapter 12

THE POWER OF PRAYER

"God's wealth is circulating in my life; his wealth flows to me in avlanches of abundance. All my needs, desires and goals are met through my faith in God and God is everything."

ANONYMOUS

The most powerful of all thoughts are prayers. Prayer is simply a conversation with God. It is a communication of thanks and praise for all the blessings of life. It gives you a time to reflect on your past and ponder your future with life's Almighty Creator. It is also a time to ask for help and seek guidance. And in prayer, you can entrust all your cares, worries and needs to a power that is personally involved in you.

Prayer is the truest connection with our spiritual world and has the force to transform and direct our energies in the most positive way. When you tell God your problems and humbly ask for help, you are submitting to a power far greater than yourself. By giving it to God, you are relinquishing the controls of your life and are allowing Him to take you in a direction that He sees best. God has constructed within all of us the power necessary for successful healthy living, and our thoughts through prayer are the mechanism to tap into this available force.

Whether or not you believe in God or a higher power, you have to agree there are unexplained energy forces working throughout the universe that affect us all. And these mighty forces can have a profound effect on our health. Medical science is now realizing the importance of prayer and its powerful effect on the healing process. In a Dartmouth Medical School study, it was found that patients are 12 times more likely to survive open-heart surgery if they have a professed faith in God and practice prayer. Also, people who attend religious services at least once a week have stronger immune systems than people who don't, concludes a Duke University medical study. It is believed the use of prayer in the religious services helps reduce stress, thereby improving the immune system.

Three out of every 10 Americans report they experienced a remarkable healing in their life, according to a Gallup poll commissioned by the Harvard Medical School. Forty-two percent of those surveyed attributed the healing to God, Jesus Christ or a higher power, while 30 percent said it was a direct result of prayer, either their own or by others. In another medical study involving prayer, sick patients were randomly divided into two different groups. One group received special prayers for their recovery from a prayer group. These sick patients were unaware they were being prayed for. The second group of sick individuals did not receive any formal prayers from this prayer group. After several months, it was concluded that the group receiving the special prayers from the prayer group recovered more quickly and more successfully than the group receiving no prayers. Quite remarkable, wouldn't you think?

In fact, the last decade has seen 30 of the nation's top medical schools institute programs to teach physicians how to tap into the patient's spiritual beliefs, which seems to promote faster healing and better health. The power of prayer is definitely starting to catch on in the medical community. Dr. Steve Caplan, an internist, organizes prayer groups for his patients in central Texas by publishing the names in the newspaper of those who request prayer for their healing. Like so many physicians, Dr. Caplan has seen prayer work many times in the lives of his patients.

During a recent conference at Harvard dealing with prayer and medicine, Dr. Caplan recalled a middle-aged female patient who entered the hospital with a severe bacterial blood infection. The woman was eventually placed on artificial life support. With almost every organ in her body failing, doctors urged the family to turn off the life support machine that was keeping her alive. But not Dr. Caplan, who, along with the family, continued to pray for the patient. Even though there was little hope of recovery, Caplan and the family never gave up prayer. Then a miracle occurred. Within six weeks after the patient hit rock bottom, she walked out of the hospital—100 percent recovered! As Dr. Caplan noted, "This was a miracle in every sense of the word. That is the power of prayer in the healing process."

Although most prayer studies involve the Christian faith, it doesn't necessarily mean they are the only ones who benefit from their spirituality. Jewish, Muslim, Buddhist and other practicing religions all receive health benefits from their faith. According to Harvard mind/body researcher Herbert Benson, MD, "It doesn't matter which god you worship or which theology you embrace, practicing a spiritual life is very healthy." So, no matter what your religious affiliation is, the power of prayer is universal.

THE SUCCESS RITUAL

There is one anchoring habit that will guarantee your success not only in your health but in other aspects of your life as well. I call it the success ritual. It requires approximately 10 to 15 minutes in the morning and about 10 minutes in the evening. The success ritual is best done in a very quiet and private area where you will not be disturbed. To start with, I recommend following the deep, diaphragmatic breathing habit described in Health Habit 12. During your deep-breathing routine, visualize a calm and peaceful scene, maybe an ocean sunset or majestic mountaintop view. Make it a very pleasant and soothing picture. It might help if you mentally repeat such relaxing words as "tranquility" or "serenity." Just the mere mention of these words brings a sense of calm.

After about four to six minutes of diaphragmatic breathing and mental imagery, practice a few moments of silence. Remain as still as possible, and try to think as little as you can. If you have noisy surroundings, I recommend earplugs. It is very important that you remain as silent and still as you can. You may continue to visualize peaceful and calming images during the suggested minutes of silent deliberation.

After practicing a few minutes of silence, I recommend reviewing and visualizing your most important written goals. By focusing on your primary goals at least twice daily, you are demonstrating persistence and faith, which are essential for their success. By painting the picture of your goals as you study them daily, you transmit the image to your subconscious mind, which ultimately drives your behavior. Write your main goals on a card as described in Health Habit 2. On the back of this card write the words "Ask and it shall be given you, seek and ye shall find, knock and it shall be opened unto you." Look at this card several times during the day, especially during your morning and evening success ritual.

SPIRITUAL CONNECTION

Now you are ready for the most important habit of all—the habit of prayer. I realize some of you may hold different spiritual beliefs than I do. So, instead of ending your success ritual with prayer, you might wish to substitute some form of meditation or personal reflection. A success ritual including mediation instead of personal prayer will still offer amazing benefits to your health and well-being.

But for the greatest value, I personally recommend prayer. Prayer allows me to clear my mind of negative energy, and it is one of the best ways to eliminate stress and worry, especially before I go to sleep (most medical experts agree that reducing stress is the most important means for improving one's health). In the Bible, it says, "If you believe, you will receive whatever you ask for in prayer."The key word here is believe. By believing, you demonstrate faith, and when you step out in faith, God will give you the success you seek. Whether it's asking to adopt a difficult habit or requesting a more peaceful and harmonious life, God hears your prayers. However, He answers our prayers in our best interest. After all, He knows better than we do what is best for us. When you talk to God always, express a willingness to accept His will. Ask for what you want, but be willing to take what God gives you. It may be better than what you ask for. As Frank Laubach put it, "Prayer is the mightiest power in the world."

The person who prays the most
accomplishes the most.

Deep breathing, silent meditation, focusing on your goals and prayer (or meditation)—all makeup the success ritual. I cannot stress enough the importance of this anchoring habit. So, please try this all-important health habit for 30 days, and I guarantee your life will never be the same.

HEALTH HABIT 2:
Write your most important health goals or desired habits on a card, and look at them as much as possible throughout the day. Review it in the

morning and in the evening before bedtime by visualizing the goal's successful accomplishment.

HEALTH HABIT 1:
Develop and follow a personal success ritual that involves deep, diaphragmatic breathing, silent meditation, visualizing your goals and prayer. Practice this success ritual in the morning and right before bedtime. It is the most important health habit you can develop.

CLOSING

All of the healthy habits in this book will benefit you very little if you don't understand the immense power of your thoughts. Self-directing your thoughts truly is the owner's manual to your mind. You do indeed become what you think about, and it is your thoughts that provide the guiding forces to maximizing your life's potential.

I hope and pray that you will benefit from this book as much as I have been blessed in preparing it for you. I sincerely thank you for your investment of time and money in this literary project. Before I close, I would like to leave you with one of my favorite quotes from Norman Vincent Peale.

"I believe that I am always divinely guided.
I believe that I will always make the right turn of the road.
And I believe God will always make a way where there is no way."

May God Richly Bless You,
Sam Varner

The 12 Habits Of Health

HEALTH HABIT 12:

Practice deep, diaphragmatic breathing at least ten minutes in the morning and ten minutes in the evening. Inhale, hold and exhale your breath for a cadence of 1 to 3 to 2. Repeat this 1-3-2 breathing cycle for a total of 10 times in the morning and 10 times in the evening. For example, if it takes you a 6 count to inhale, then hold your filled lungs for an 18 count (6 times 3) and exhale through your mouth for a 12 count (6 times 2).

HEALTH HABIT 11:

Drink a full glass (10 to 12 ounces) of filtered water before every meal and snack, and before and after all exercise.

HEALTH HABIT 10:

Drink approximately 12 to 24 ounces of warm water with fresh lemon juice from half a lemon upon arising every morning.

HEALTH HABIT 9:

Eat adequate low-fat protein sources such as fish, chicken, turkey, eggs, cottage cheese, beef and plain yogurt daily. The amount of dietary protein intake should be specific and individualized for your lean body weight and activity level. See Figure 6.1 in Chapter 6 to calculate your lean weight and activity level.

HEALTH HABIT 8:

Consume a fresh green salad or fibrous vegetable with every meal except breakfast. Fresh green garden salads are probably the healthiest food you can consume. Fibrous vegetables include asparagus, broccoli, lettuce, carrots, celery, cucumber, spinach, artichokes, cabbage, cauliflower, kale, mushrooms, sprouts, peppers and tomatoes. Also include onions and garlic regularly.

HEALTH HABIT 7:

Consume fresh fruit with breakfast and as a snack. Eat fresh fruits in their whole, natural state. Recommended fresh fruits are apples, apricots, berries, cantaloupe, cherries, grapefruit, grapes, melon, kiwi, nectarines, oranges, peaches, pears, pineapple, plums, tangerines and watermelon.

HEALTH HABIT 6:

Minimize or avoid processed carbohydrate consumption such as white breads, plain pasta, sweets, pastries, muffins, candy, sugary drinks, soda pop, chips, processed cereals and cookies.

HEALTH HABIT 5:

Wake up and go to sleep at the same time every day and achieve at least eight hours of sleep every 24 hours, weekends included. Even if you stay up later than usually, always awaken at the same time. Abstain from food or drink for two to three hours prior to your normal bedtime.

HEALTH HABIT 4:

Do some form of aerobic or movement exercise at least five days a week, striving for 30 minutes in duration. Movements such as walking, jogging, hiking, dancing, playing games, biking, swimming and walking your pet are just a few examples. Your goal is to break a sweat or at least get a little out of breath.

HEALTH HABIT 3:

Do 15 to 60 minutes of weight training or resistance exercises at least two times per week.

HEALTH HABIT 2:

Write your most important health goals or desired habits on a card, and look at them as much as possible throughout the day. Review it in the morning and in the evening before bedtime by visualizing the goal's successful accomplishment.

HEALTH HABIT 1:

Develop and follow a personal success ritual that involves deep, diaphragmatic breathing, silent meditation, visualizing your goals and prayer. Practice this success ritual in the morning and right before bedtime. It is the most important health habit you can develop.

Slimmer, Younger, Stronger Favorite Recipes

SAM'S GARDEN GREEN TURKEY SALAD

Ingredients:

2 cups romaine lettuce

2 medium celery stalks

1/4 of a medium peeled cucumber

1/8 cup of red onion

1 small ripe tomato

8 ounces of turkey breast

Juice from 1/4 of a lemon

1/4 cup of your favorite dressing (I recommend honey mustard or blue cheese. Don't use nonfat of low-fat dressing)

Salt

Pepper

Preparation Time: 10 minutes

Finely chop romaine, celery, cucumber, onion, tomato and turkey breast and thoroughly mix together in a large bowl. Add lemon juice, 2 to 4 tablespoons or your favorite salad dressing. Add a dash of salt and pepper to taste. Serves 2 to 3.

SAM'S SPECIAL CHICKEN CAESAR'S SALAD

Ingredients:

2 cups romaine lettuce

2 medium celery stalks

1/4 cup of red onion

3 garlic cloves

1 small ripe tomato

2 chicken breasts

Juice from 1/4 of a lemon

1/4 cup of olive oil

3/4 cup of Caesar's Dressing

1/4 cup Parmesan cheese

Salt

Pepper

Preparation time: 10 minutes

Cooking time: 10 to 12 minutes

Cut chicken breast into small, 1/2 inch pieces and marinate in 1/2 cup of Caesar's dressing for at least 20 minutes. Finely chop romaine, celery, tomato, and mix together in large mixing bowl. Also, finely chop onion and garlic but do not mix with other salad ingredients. Heat 1/4 cup of olive oil in wok. Stir in marinated chicken pieces. Stir chicken until all pink color has disappeared. Add onion and garlic. Cook until chicken becomes golden brown. Cover, turn off heat, and let the wok ingredients cool. Pour wok ingredients into salad bowl with other salad ingredients and thoroughly mix. Add lemon juice, 1/4 cup of Caesar's dressing and Parmesan cheese. Mix again. Add a dash of salt and pepper to taste. Serves 2 to 3.

SAM'S BAKED BAY SEASONED SALMON

Ingredients:

2 pounds of fresh salmon

Bay Seasoning

2 lemons

Preparation time: 10 minutes

Cooking time: 40 minutes

Preheat oven to 350°. Cut salmon into 4-ounce strips. (2 pounds yields 8 strips.) Place each salmon strip separately onto 8"by 12"aluminum foil section. Sprinkle approximately 1/2 teaspoon of Bay Seasoning over salmon. Squeeze juice from 1/4 lemon onto salmon strip and leave lemon wedge on salmon. Wrap fish and lemon slice in aluminum foil and place on cooking sheet. Cook salmon strips for 40 minutes at 350°. Let salmon strips cool. Put them in air-tight container and then place them in the refrigerator. To eat, simply remove salmon from aluminum foil and heat it in the microwave for approximately 45 seconds. Yields 8 servings.

PARMESAN ONION OMELETTE

Ingredients:

2 Egg Beaters or 4 large egg whites
1/4 cup minced onions
1/8 cup of Parmesan cheese
1/4 cup of olive oil

Preparation time: 8 minutes
Cooking time: 5 minutes

Sauté onions in olive oil on medium-high heat. Add whipped eggs followed by Parmesan cheese. Cook until eggs are desired texture. Then fold omelette. Serves 2. For added flavor, serve with salsa.

MARINATED TEQUILA CHICKEN

(WITHOUT THE WORM)

Ingredients:

2 chicken breasts

1 shot of tequila

1/4 cup of lime juice

Preparation time: 25 minutes

Cooking time: 30 minutes

Marinate chicken breasts in tequila and lime juice for approximate 20 minutes. Then broil for about 30 minutes or until golden brown. Serve with sauteed vegetables or steamed broccoli with cheddar cheese. Serves 2.

BAKED HERB CHICKEN

Ingredients:

2 chicken breasts

1/2 teaspoon parsley

1/2 teaspoon rosemary

1/2 teaspoon tarragon

1/2 teaspoon oregano

Juice from 1/4 lemon

Preparation time: 8 minutes

Cooking time: 45 minutes

Preheat oven to 350°. Wrap chicken breasts in aluminum foil with herbs and lemon juice. Bake for 45 minutes at 350°.

MARINATED BRANDY HALIBUT

Ingredients:

1 pound of fresh halibut

1/4 cup brandy

1/2 cup apricot juice

Preparation time: 10 minutes

Cooking time: 40 minutes

Preheat oven to 350°. Cut halibut into 4 ounce portions and marinate in brandy and apricot juice for at least 20 minutes. Then place marinated fish into baking dish and bake for 40 minutes at 350°. Serve with tossed green salad or sauteed zucchini slice. Serves 4.

SAM'S TOSSED TUNA SALAD

Ingredients:

2 cup iceberg lettuce (or romaine lettuce)

1 large tomato

1 medium avocado

2 medium celery stalks

1/2 large peeled cucumber

Two 6-ounce cans of drained white albacore tuna in spring water

Juice from 1/2 lemon

1/3 cup of Miracle Whip or mayonnaise

Salt

Pepper

Preparation time: 10 minutes

Finely chop lettuce, celery, cucumber, tomato, avocado and mix together in large bowl with tuna. Add lemon juice and salad dressing (Miracle Whip or mayonnaise). Mix thoroughly. Add a dash of salt and pepper to taste. Serves 4 to 5.

About the Author

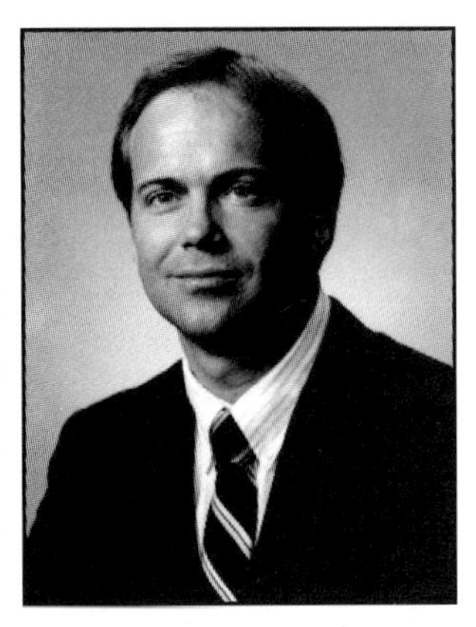

Sam Varner was born and raised in North Carolina and received degrees in biology and food science-nutrition from North Carolina State University in 1978. From 1979 to 1982, he was a strength and conditioning coach for the Clemson University football team that included an undefeated National Championship team and a victory in the 1982 Orange Bowl. He also served two stints as strength and conditioning coach for the University of Utah athletic program between 1982 to 1990. Sam was certified as a strength and conditioning specialist (CSCS) in 1985 by the National Strength and Condition Association. After his first stint at Utah, Sam joined the United States Ski team staff in the same capacity where he trained seven Olympic medalists, Picabo Street, Tommy Moe, Hilary Lindh, Kyle Rassmussen, Debbie Armstrong, Diane Roffe and Bill Johnson. He has worked on the staff of three national coaches of the year, which include Rick Majerus, former head basketball coach of the University of Utah; Jim Fassel, former head football coach of the New York Giants; and Danny Ford, former head football coach of Clemson University. Sam has also been a very successful personal trainer to many athletes and celebrities such as actress Faye Dunaway; John Kacinski, 1994 and 1997 World Champion Superbike Motorcycle Racer; Scott Mitchell, former NFL quarterback; and Ed Ames, former costar on the Daniel Boone television series. He currently conducts health and motivational seminars, writes freelance articles, and is working on his next book. If you would like to contact Sam, visit www.cliffscommunities.com for information.

References

Allen, J. *As A Man Thinketh*, Putnam Publishing Group, 1959.

Andrews, S. S., L. A. Balart, C. B. Morrison and H. L. Steward, *Sugar Busters*, Ballantine Publishing Group, 1995.

Appleton, N. *Lick the Sugar Habit*, Avery Publishing Group, 1996.

Atkins, R. *Dr. Atkins' Diet Revolution*, Bantam Books, 1972.

Audette, R. Neanderthin: *A Cave Man's Guide to Nutrition*, Paleolithic Press, 1995.

Bailey, C. *Smart Exercise*, Houghton Mifflin Company, 1994.

Burton Goldberg Group, *Alternative Medicine*, Future Medicine Publishing, 1993.

Cassidy, C. *Research from Smithsonian Institute*, 1980.

Chopra, C. *Restful Sleep*, Harmony Books, 1994.

Conkling, W. "Water," *American Health*, May 1995.

Coren, S. *Sleep Thieves*, The Free Press, 1996.

Donsbach, K. "Cholesterol," International Institute of Natural Health Sciences, 1977.

Eades, M. R. and M. D. Eades, *Protein Power*, Bantam Books, 1996.

Emerson, R. W. *Selective Writings of Ralph Waldo Emerson*, Penguin Books, 1965.

Erasmus, U. *Fats That Heal, Fats That Kill*, Alive Books, 1986, 1993.

Franklin, B. *Poor Richard's Almanac*, Reprint Services Corp., 1993.

Goldblatt, H. *Journal of Experimental Medicine*, 1934, 59: 347-379.

Helm, M. "Wake Up and Get More Sleep," *Hearst Newspapers*, March 3, 1998.

Henderson, C. E. "Suggestion: Formulation and Application," Biocentrix, 1980.

Hendricks, G. *Conscious Breathing: Breathwork for Health, Stress, Release, and Personal Mastery*, Bantam Books, 1993.

Hill, J. and J. Peters, *Science*, 280:1371--1373, 1998.

Hill, N. *Think and Grow Rich*, Fawcett Crest, Ballantine Books, 1960.

Inlander, C. B. and C. K. Moran, *67 Ways to Good Sleep*, Walker and Company, 1995.

Jenner, B. *Finding the Champion Within*, Simon and Schuster, 1996.

Lee, K. "Outrun Destiny," *Health Magazine*, September 1998.

Levine, B. In a statement issued by Nutrition Information Center, New York Hospital–Cornell Medical Center, May 1998.

Maas, J. *Power Sleep*, Villard Books, 1998.

Millman, D. *The Laws of Spirit: Simple, Powerful Truths for Making Life Work*, H. J. Kramer, 1995.

Mosby's Medical Encyclopedia, Mosby-Year Book, TLC Properties, 1997.

Netzer, C. T. *The Complete Book of Food Counts*, Dell Publishing, 1991.

Nightingale, E. *Earl Nightingale's Greatest Discovery*, Dodd, Mead and Company, Inc, 1987.

Nightingale, E. *Life's Strangest Secret*, Keys Company, 1956, 1997.

Peale, N. V. *The Power Of Positive Thinking*, Prentice-Hall, Inc., 1952.

Perkes, K. S. "Medical Study Finds People Heal Faster If They Practice Religion," Living Section of *Monterey County Herald*, March 28, 1998.

Physician's Desk Reference, Medical Economics Company, 1999, p. 1666-1667.

Rimm, E. B. and W. C. Willett, "Folate and Vitamin B-6 From Diet and Supplements in Relation to Risk of Coronary Heart Disease Among Women," *Journal of the American Medical Association*, February 4, 1998, 279: 359-364.

Robb, J. *The Fat Burning Diet*, Loving Health Publications, 1994.

Robbins, A. "Personal Power," Robbins Research International, Guthy-Renker Corporation, 1993.

Rosenbloom, C. "Living Longer, Living Better," Georgia State University, October 8, 1998.

Rowe, J. W. and R. L. Kahn, *Successful Aging*, Pantheon Books, 1998.

Ryan, M. "Sometimes It's Good to Nap on the Job," *Parade Magazine*, March 22, 1998, p. 16.

Schnakenberg, D. In a statement issued by American Society of Clinical Nutrition, 1998.

Sears, B. *The Zone*, HarperCollins, 1995.

Shields, J. W. "Lymph, Lymph Glands, and Homeostasis," *Lymphology Journal*, 25, no. 4, December 1992.

The American College of Cardiology, "Preventing Heart Disease," *Prevention Magazine*, December 1998.

The Life Recovery Bible, *The Living Bible*, Tyndale House Publishers, Inc., 1992.

Weil, A. *Health and Healing*, Houghton Mifflin, 1988.

Weil, A. *The Natural Mind*, Houghton Mifflin, 1972.

Zi, N. *The Art of Breathing*, Bantam Books, 1986